The
Healing
Power
of Clay

The Healing Power of Clay

The Natural Remedy for Dozens of Common Ailments

Michel Abehsera

CITADEL PRESS
Kensington Publishing Corp.
www.kensingtonbooks.com

CITADEL PRESS BOOKS are published by

Kensington Publishing Corp.
850 Third Avenue
New York, NY 10022

All Kensington titles, imprints, and distributed lines are available at special quantity discounts for bulk purchases for sales promotions, premiums, fund-raising, educational, or institutional use. Special book excerpts or customized printings can also be created to fit specific needs. For details, write or phone the office of the Kensington special sales manager: Kensington Publishing Corp., 850 Third Avenue, New York, NY 10022, attn: Special Sales Department, phone 1-800-221-2647.

Citadel Press and the Citadel Logo are trademarks of Kensington Publishing Corp.

First Kensington printing: November 2001

10 9 8 7 6 5 4 3

Printed in the United States of America

Library of Congress Control Number: 2001092762

ISBN 0-8065-1942-8

Foreword

Only three years ago clay was an unknown curing agent. There have always been those who used it - for years, perhaps, but the cure remained their own and never spread beyond their local region. It seems that those who used it did not dare to publicize "mud" as an alternative cure. In Morocco where I was born we also had such primitive cures which we kept to ourselves, thinking that they would never be accepted by the modern world.

Almost every child knew how to stop bleeding if he happened to cut himself in the woods, until the time came when modern means of cure forced themselves on us. We exchanged the old for the new unknowingly. Who would have guessed then that that which is modern is almost always full of many chemical substances alien to the body and therefore often harmful to health. Some of us intuitively were aware of the risk we were running; nevertheless, we went for the adventure. The modern way seemed arrogantly clean and fast-working, compared to the primitive way which then seemed slow-working and demanded attention and knowledge on our part. Natural medicine involves the whole of the person; the patient cannot merely sit back and rest, waiting to be acted upon. There must be participation, and decisions must be made. One must actively choose the cure; this demands some thinking, whereas in modern medicine, you let the other think for you. It is an unfortunate play of circumstances where, with time, one loses contact with the most obvious means of cure. The fear of having to choose which medicine to take is so great that one slides deeper and deeper into the belief that the best and most practical cure is the modern one since it responds quickly to people's ills. 'If it is made for and by humans', he thinks, 'used by millions, it is certainly good for me. If it is bad, it's bad for all of us. Why should I be an exception?'

That is roughly the general attitude of those who prefer to overeat and then take a medical prescription rather than toning down their wants with a thoughtful way of eating. To do that demands some sacrifices on the sensorial side; no more is he a person eating with the senses of a young lad full of desires for delicious things no matter how they were made, but a whole man who eats for completeness of himself and not fullness of his belly.

The ability to control oneself at the table demonstrates maturity. That one act of control is proof that in everything we do we will be able to do it with moderation. Imagine, then, someone who eats without end-he will constantly direct all his energies towards that one goal-food-until it becomes the overriding force in his life.

It is there fore best to be moderate and not be swayed to either extreme. There are people whose conversation consists almost entirely of healthy eating. This is an attitude which often borders on paranoia. Being always on the alert about food may lead one to dislike those who do not eat healthily. Adhering to moderation in one's desires is wise. It gives a person the opportunity to see things clearly until the time he reaches the point where what he really needs in order to grow becomes obvious. From this plateau one can fast without harm, and can also eat much at a happy gathering without feeling bad about it, or from it.

Much of the material here is gathered from the works of Raymond Dextreit, the French naturopath. It is thanks to him that I came to learn the wondrous workings of clay. Mr. Dextreit is perhaps the most popular and most read naturopath in his country, where he has made the clay treatment well known. The volume of grateful correspondence that he receives from people who have been helped testifies to the excellence of his medicine.

Mr. Dextreit's medicine is simple to use, yet it demanded great research and long practice on his part. Over thirty years of dedication with millions of books bought are the best proof. In *Our Earth, Our Cure* he displays an amazing knowledge of the difficult field of medicine. Some might disagree with the all-vegetarian stand of Mr. Dextreit; notwithstanding, the English version of his work. *Our Earth, Our Cure* is a must if one wishes to study the organism's human organism.

The present book also contains new material that I gleaned here and there from different sources as well as from personal experience.

The reader should not be wary about using clay as medicine. It would be proper to read what follows before making a hasty judgment one way or the other about clay.

May what follows serve for the most excellent purpose of alleviating the pains of all suffering people everywhere.

The Author.

Note

I am serving as a reporter in this book on the wonders of clay. I do not claim to be a "clay-healer"; I am just one among the many who experienced the benefits of clay and wishes to make it known to others. Everything I know about the amazing clay is contained in this small book; that frees me from the obligation to answer all inquiries that anyone would wish to make.

The reader should know that I am not a doctor and therefore could not possibly give any prescriptions of any sort.

CONTENTS

Chapter 1
THE WONDERS OF CLAY

This small book became necessary when many people expressed the desire for the clay cure to be put in a short and practical form. The book *Our Earth, Our Cure* includes the clay cure; however, not everyone wants a book on vegetarianism when he is only interested in the clay cure. Furthermore this book is an updated edition about the wonders of clay. It is more complete and organized in such a way that the reader can quickly and easily find what he is looking for.

One does not necessarily have to be a strict vegetarian to benefit from clay. Anyone willing to try it will experience results; however, only a methodical way of eating will help bring about permanent results.

A vegetarian of course gets the best out of it, for the purpose of both clay and fruits and vegetables are the same—to 'cleanse' and purify the organism, especially the blood. Eating too many starches, white breads, large amounts of meat, cheese, cakes and other clogging agents do not let clay work at its best. Most diseases start from poor nourishment of the organs; the blood is so thick and full of waste that the organism is only partially active because of the various obstructions that take place as a consequence.

A good and balanced diet should aim at keeping the blood fluid enough to allow good circulation. Most diseases will not take a firm hold of any part of the body as long as there is good blood circulation. The vegetarian is very conscious of that; he always eats with this idea in mind.

A good blood circulation could very well be assured by following a diet that is not as restrictive as strict vegetarianism. If one goes overboard at times it is best to resume eating more wisely whatever is best for him—fruits, vegetables or grains. It is good to make room for forms of cure other than constantly concentrating on cleansing and purifying. This is a detrimental attitude which limits one's field of action. To do so is to not allow the many wonders of this world to take place. Everything is so restricted to cleansing that the aim of life becomes that and that alone. One then expects everything to happen through the vegetarian channel.

This does not give license to a person freeing himself from the obligation to purify himself with food under the pretext that it is too involving. Both attitudes are extreme; one would rather get sick than give up his heavy meat-eating habit and the other develops the fear of anything else but what his diet permits.

The golden rule is to reach an equilibrium which is neither conceptual nor a sensorial compromise. A balance is not an intellectual decision, it is rather a healthy frame of mind that is acquired with time. It is formed by various factors. The most important of them is being fully aware of his goal in life. When a person is socially and spiritually active, helping others, one comes to forget to be so sensitive to *things* around one. Caring for another human being makes one forget oneself a bit, and this is a higher form of health.

If in the course of the book it should happen that the reader is urged to be strict in his manner of eating—and this for a long while, having nothing else but grains, vegetables and some fruits—this would not in any way contradict what was written previously. One has to start somewhere; strictness in the observance of a diet is the best possible way to the cure. We cannot be philosophical about it or too lenient to gain the approval of the reader. When disease occurs one should leave it to Nature to do its work. There is nothing lowly about this, as long as one is cognizant of the fact that all cures and miracles come from the Owner of this world.

Chapter 2
THE HEALING SECRET

Clay has been used for thousands of years and yet no one has been able to pin down what makes it a healer. A naturopath asks only that it should heal; he does not delve into details. He is too happy to use it in every case he judges appropriate and achieve good results. That is why he is full of wonder every time clay accomplishes a cure that he did not expect to happen in so little time. Most of the users of clay leave scientific explanations aside when they become astounded by the accomplishments of clay. Some of the scientists who ventured in the search for clues to the secret of clay found a number of minerals such as: silica, aluminum, magnesium, titanium, iron, calcium, sodium, potassium, manganese, and others. The presence of a mineral can justify a few cures; however, when clay deeply affects several diseases of opposite natures, the main explanation must be found elsewhere than in the mere mineral content of clay.

Many hypotheses have been suggested and many of them contribute to giving some rational explanations to clay's miracles. However they are far from satisfying as to the real factor of cure.

Raymond Dextreit, the French naturopath who popularized the clay cure in his country, says the following: "One of clay's peculiarities is based on its physical-chemical domination. From a thermodynamic point of view, we must admit that clay cannot be the sole source of energy of the phenomena it produces. Clay is effective as a dynamic presence far more significantly than a mere consideration of the substances it contains. It is a catalyst rather than an agent itself. This is possible because clay is alive."

Louis Kervran, the French scientist, world-famous for his provocative work on Biological Transmutations, writes about a shrimp that lives in clay: "It has been known for a long time that living organisms inhabit clay without any organic supply of food from the outside. This fact has intrigued research workers . . . Note the case of the Niphargus shrimp, a small animal half-an-inch long that lives in the clay of caves. If a shrimp is given organic matter such as meat, it vegetates and dies. It also dies if it is not kept in humid clay. Experiments have shown that it grows normally in pure clay to which nothing has been added. Research workers therefore thought that the shrimp lived on clay and nothing but clay, an impossibility according to the laws of biochemistry. Actually, it cannot live thus in clay alone, but this clay contains microorganisms which work for the shrimp, making vitamins, various mineral products, nitrogen, phosphorus, and calcium, etc."

Clay then is a live medium which helps generate and maintain life. Dextreit says on this subject: "Among the properties to which we can attribute the effect of clay is radioactivity. Clay is radioactive to a degree but this radioactivity is generally imperceptible to the testing apparatus used in laboratories at present . . . Radioesthetically the matter has been extensively discussed. Scientists differ widely as to the significance of this radioactivity in clay.

7

The problem is further complicated by the differences between one clay and another."

It seems that clay has, among other properties, the ability to either stimulate a deficiency or absorb an excess in the radioactivity of the body on which it is applied. On an organism which has suffered and still retains the radiations of radium or any other intensive radioactive source, the radioactivity is first enhanced and then absorbed. A clay could, in this way, ensure the protection of an organism overexposed to atomic radiations. This radioactive effect has been laboratory tested; today, when everyone is forcibly submitted to many artificially provoked radioactive substances, such as dust in the atmosphere from bomb testing, everything increasing this danger should be avoided. Experiments made with the Geiger counter have demonstrated that dry clay absorbs a very important part of this surrounding activity.

Clay's therapeutic powers are certainly enhanced by radioactivity, however, this also does not explain all the wondrous cures it provides. More people—scientists and laymen—became fascinated with it and some looked for more clues to its healing powers. They provide some minimal explanation—just enough to whet one's curiosity and interest for this peculiarly fine earth.

Clay has a negative electrical attraction for particles that are positively charged. In the organism most of the toxic poisons are positively charged. These toxins are irresistibly drawn towards the clay. Moreover, according to an authority on Bentonite (another name for the energetic clay) "clay's particles being shaped like a 'calling card' with the wide surfaces negative and the edges of the card positive, have many times more negative than positive pulling power."

The same authority writes the following: "the very minuteness of the particles of Bentonite gives a large surface area in proportion to the volume used, thus enabling it to pick up many times its weight in positively charged particles." According to Robert T. Martin, B.S., University of Minnesota, Ph.D., Cornell University, and Mineralogist at Massachusetts Institute of Technology, one gram of this product has a surface area of 800 square meters. The greater the surface area the greater its power to pick up positively charged particles.

The same report which quotes Dr. Martin gives an important statement that every user of clay is aware of: that "to obtain maximum effectiveness in the human body, it should be put in a liquid colloidal-gel state. This is why it cannot be made into tablet form."*

A quote from an edition of the Dispensatory of the United States of America says the following: "In aqueous suspensions, the individual particles of Bentonite are negatively charged, thus resulting in a strong attraction for positively charged particles and being responsible for the ability of Bentonite to clarify such liquid as contains positively charged particles of suspended matter. . . . . In addition to the growing number of external uses for Bentonite, it has been reported to be of value as an intestinal evacuant when in the form of a gel."

The same study on Bentonite gives no evidence that it has any chemical effect on the organism. Its actions seem to be purely physical. This throws a bit more light on the phenomenon of clay. The rectangular shape of the clay particles keep it in maximum potency. If, for example, the

*Dextreit states further on, however, that it is possible to dry small clay balls and swallow them whole. This is true for the green clay of which he speaks and may also be for others as well.

particles would have been round, not much energy could be retained or passed on, as anything round does not have the edges needed to receive and pass on energy. The angular shape of its particles allows a constant interplay of energies in the give-and-take process. The existing radioactivity makes the interplay between the negative and positive poles of the particles very potent. It may be this constant switching from negative to positive charges that makes the clay a healing agent for so many different types of diseases. As Dextreit writes: "The same teaspoon of clay can cure an obstinate carbuncle and tenacious anemia equally well. Curing the carbuncle is explained by clay's absorbent power . . . but anemia?!"

One marvels at what clay can do. We would not go as far as to label it a cure-all; however, it remains that for something that looks to be merely an inert matter, it gives quite a performance.

Absorbent Action

The absorbent power of clay is extraordinary. According to Dextreit, raw eggs covered with clay lose three times more weight than if they remained in the open air, without causing any damage to the eggshell.

When clay is used as a body deodorant, or when foul-smelling substances are mixed with clay, the odor disappears, absorbed by the clay. If clay is placed in the bottom of the bed pan of an invalid the evacuations will be completely deodorized.

Clay has the power to attract and either absorb or stimulate the evacuation of toxic and non-useful elements. In general, clay has remarkable resistance to chemical agents and only the most energetic ones can attack it. As a bacteria-destroying agent it can render contaminated water innocuous. Its absorbent power has contributed to the elimination of the chemical taste of chloride in Paris water. This action is not limited to deodorization but when ingested, it travels along the digestive path and uproots many unwelcome intrusive bodies, including gas.

Raymond Dextreit brings out that clay's absorbent power is so great that if it is put in a place where water has been stagnating to the point of emitting a bad smell, the foul odor vanishes in a relatively short time.

Clay is particularly rich in certain diastases and enzymes which do not destroy themselves in action. Some of these diastases, the *oxidases,* have the power of fixing free oxygen, which explains the purifying and enriching action of clay in the blood.

The knowledge of these properties would be insufficient to explain clay's active power if we did not already know that clay is a powerful agent of stimulation, transformation and transmission of energy. As every filing which comes from a magnet keeps its properties, every piece of clay retains a considerable amount of energy from the large and powerful magnetic entity of the Earth. This radioactive action transmits an extraordinary strength to the organism and helps to rebuild vital potential through the liberation of latent energy. The organism has great energy resources which normally remain dormant; clay awakens them.

Absorbent Powers

All that was previously said still does not completely explain the multiple actions of clay. One can only tell of all the various wonders it accomplishes.

Raymond Dextreit praises its absorbent and adsorbent powers: absorption of the impurities in the tissues, neutralizing and draining these impurities. Adsorption means the pulling out of the impurities that are in a state of suspension in the body liquid (blood, lymph, bile) and then draining and eliminating them. It is precisely these properties of clay which cause its use in the hundreds of thousands of tons in the petroleum industry, purification of gasoline and other industries, especially in margarine processing, to deodorize some of the raw materials. It is also used in the processing of medicinal oils.

Clay considerably reduces the toxicity of harmful substances. Dextreit relates a famous incident that happened in France in which dogs had been poisoned, but survived, thanks to the clay which had been put in their drinking water.

The nutritionist Linda Clark mentions in her recent book, *The Best of Linda Clark,* that a European doctor, Meyer-Camberg, recommends clay for neutralizing poisons. According to Dr. Meyer-Camberg, clay takes care of any bad poisoning such as arsenic! It suffices to take 1 teaspoonful of clay mixed in a glass of water every hour for six hours to be out of trouble.

Dextreit is certain of the antiseptic and antibiotic powers of clay, but it puzzles him. As with all natural remedies, clay does not act specifically on one or several bacteria varieties; rather it prevents their proliferation by reinforcing the defenses of the organism. Acting in all directions, the good earth sometimes slows down the bowel movement, creating a temporary constipation. In this case, it is best to complement its action with a laxative herb decoction such as buckthorn, senna, rhubarb, etc.

It may happen that some of these properties take time to manifest themselves; notwithstanding, its revitalizing effects are often spectacular. It is thanks to these vital and energetic properties that the organism is put in the best conditions of defense.

The other side of the coin is that the revitalization is sometimes so energetic that it may be accompanied by a state of nervous excitation. That which is latent becomes manifest. Natural remedies always lead to the exteriorization of symptoms. It is one of the surest means of diagnosis.

Contributing to the neutralization of the nitrogenized wastes and to the elimination of acids clay favors a good pH of the blood, one which is slightly alkaline. If the organism of the vegetarian does not succumb to disease, it is because of his diet which is predominantly composed of alkaline substances, creating a delicate equilibrium which is constantly renewed on account of the production of acids from the muscular activities of the organism and also by the transformation of nitrogenous wastes into acids.

It also seems from experience that clay is a catalyst,

that it favors the transformations and operations of synthesis, thus allowing a better use of the absorbed elements.

As was said previously, the above does not make of clay a cure-all medicine. It is known to have these properties; however, this does not mean that they will reproduce on anyone, at anytime. It might just not happen, and there are many reasons for this which will become obvious in the course of the book. Clay is one medicine; there are various other means of cure that should be investigated instead of putting one's trust in clay alone.

Clay in History

How has this healing power of clay been ignored for so long? Or has it been? When we look back in time we discover that clay has been used for thousands of years by many people who put all their confidence in its results.

The Egyptians used it for the mummification of their dead because they knew of its purifying powers. It is therefore nearly certain its use was not only reserved for the dead.

The doctors of antiquity did not hesitate to make use of it and many, such as the Greek Dioscorides, attributed an 'extraordinary strength' to the vital properties of clay. Long before this, the 'Prince of the Doctors,' the Arab Avicena, and the Greek anatomist, Galen, used it widely, mentioning it in terms of praise. The Roman naturalist Pliny the Elder devoted a whole chapter of his 'Natural History' to it.

The tendency of many is to assume that these ancient peoples used clay only because they lacked the other and more active medications available to us today. However, the reputation of clay has been restored, while at the same time deficiencies in the treatment of ill people by the use of drugs and chemicals has been revealed. The great German naturopaths Kneipp, Kuhn, Just, Felke and others of the last century have contributed to this revival of the use of clay in the framework of natural treatments.

The priest Kneipp strongly advised a mixture of clay and natural vinegar for packs and poultices. In some western countries this method had survived but was applied mainly to animals—when one was seriously ill, it would be daubed with a paste made of clay and vinegar.

At the end of his life, Kneipp transmitted valuable observations on clay to Adolph Just; under his direction, the clay treatment was widely extended and the Earth of Just, called 'Luvos', was soon known and appreciated. In the early part of this century, a Berlin doctor, Professor Julius Stumpf, used it successfully in the treatment of Asiatic cholera.

During the First World War, the Russian soldiers received 200 grams of it along with their rations and it was added to mustard in several French regiments, who remained free of the dysentery which ravaged nearby regiments.

In villages which we call 'primitive' because they still live in close contact with nature, the use of clay is common. All around the world can be found people and even whole tribes who eat earth . . . in Mexico, in India (Mahatma Gandhi advised the use of clay), in Anglo-Egyptian Sudan, in South America, or among the High Orinoco villages of the Cassiquare, of the Meta and Rio Negro; they knead the earth in balls or lumps and then dry and bake them when they wish to eat them.

In Switzerland and Germany doctors made use of it and in Davos, an important center for the treatment of tuberculosis, patients were usually treated with clay; the whole thorax was daubed with a paste of very hot clay and this pack was kept on all night. This treatment frequently was credited with miraculous healing.

Under the name of 'Cutler's earth,' clay was used in some districts of France—and perhaps it is still used—as a resolutive and against burns from first to third degree. It is also known under the names of Luvos, aluminum silicate, colloidal white clay, balus, and others.

More recently, its use for therapeutic purposes has been extended in France in such a way that it is impossible to argue about its properties. Recent experiments have treated sores and ulcers with aluminum; not only is clay in a great part formed by aluminum silicate, but its healing action is increased due to the fact that its components are in a state of natural dosage.

Scientific experience has now also embraced the use of previously disdained substances such as marshy mud. Those 'biogenic stimulants' applied on the skin or even to the cornea of the eye are sometimes products taken from marshy mud. These muds contain highly active ingredients, able to induce cellular rebuilding and to hasten all organic processes. This problem of rejuvenation is only solved with the help of life's resources—Nature and its elements—rather than with synthetic products.

Any similarity between clay and chemical medicine is only apparent. There is a basic difference between clay and chemical antiseptic actions. Any chemical product is a dead substance which acts blindly and destroys all bacteria indiscriminately; the good and the bad, the healthy and the ill, the useful and the harmful. It is possible for the dangerous germs to get extinguished, but the reconstructive elements are not respected and the treated tissues of sores and ulcers are reproduced in a much slower time than those not treated.

Scientists are trying to find out what is responsible for the healing value in mineral waters. They have tried to rebuild a synthetic water, using the chemical composition of the mineral waters. An amount of water has been reactivated, drawn out after a certain period of time sufficient to make it lose its radioactivity. All these experiments have failed.

Observation of nature convinces one that duplicating its properties through chemical or physical means is impossible. Chemistry and physics cannot rebuild life. This is a fact which many methods of modern science ignores. We must humbly recognize the existence of many unsolvable problems for mere man. We must observe, verify, take note and admit. We must accept the facts even if we do not understand their origin. And clay does act with wisdom—it goes to the unhealthy spot. Used internally, whether absorbed orally, anally or vaginally, clay goes to the place where harm is, there it lodges, perhaps for several days, until finally it draws out the pus, black blood, etc. with its evacuation.

From helping to prevent the proliferation of pathogenic germs and parasites to aiding with rebuilding of healthy tissues and cells, clay is a 'living' cure.

Over seventeen years ago the doctor who was treating me finally agreed to send me to Chatel-Guyen, a small town long known for its healing waters. Every day at certain hours prescribed by a local doctor people would go to various springs at different times depending on their condition. I must say that it did help me a lot even without having to greatly change my eating habits.

Along with drinking the waters every day, I would get an 'earth' treatment, which consisted of mud freshly dug, and heated so that when applied, it burned the skin even though the nurse who applied this poultice made sure to place a folded towel between the skin and the burning mud. After three weeks I was a new person. No more amoeba, dysentery or any gastro-intestinal trouble.

The trouble came back the year after that but for various reasons I was prevented from returning to this pleasant place in France.

I had had similar dramatic cures in a relatively short time. It was in the French Riviera where the sun always shines that it happened. Not having the patience nor the means to prepare proper nourishment I had recourse to quick expedients such as milk, bananas and flakes of different sorts with occasional cooked vegetables such as eggplant, green pepper and zucchini. All of these would have made me sicker than I was were I not in the south near the sea shore.

Everyday I would go to an isolated place on the beach and intuitively would cover myself with the hot sand up to my neck, remaining thus sometimes more than an hour. After three weeks of this improvised treatment I was completely relieved of the stomach and intestinal problem that I had suffered from the previous year in Paris.

Three years ago after I had already been acquainted with Raymond Dextreit's work I received a telephone call from a woman who was alone and very sick from severe intestinal pains, so much so that she could not move. She had nothing to cure herself with, except that she lived right on a beach. I remembered what hot sand had done for me. It was raining where she was, so I suggested that she gather some of the sand into a large bowl and heat it in the oven. She applied it on the abdomen two or three times and was healed. Later, through Dextreit's work and other sources I learned of the earth and sand baths which I had successfully used myself. Now when I mention these baths I am often told it is a common cure, as old as antiquity.

The Sand Cure

Of everyone who has lain on sandy beaches, exposed to the sun's rays, how many know that the sand on which they were resting is as beneficial as the sun or sea? We could profit more from its beneficial influence by covering ourselves with it—that is, by taking a true sand bath.

It is known that sand, especially marine sand, can contain certain radioactive substances, particularly Uranium. This partially explains its wonderful action on osseous afflictions. Rickets, weakness, decalcification, all troubles of the osseous system such as arthritis, rheumatism, lumbago, nephritis, sciatica and many other illnesses are helped with sand treatment.

These baths are taken in the sunshine with dry sand; dig a little so that the body is well-buried, and then cover with a thick cover of sand, leaving out only the head, which will be under the shade of foliage or an umbrella or cloth, placed at least a yard away from the head, so as to permit air circulation and avoid a concentration of heat.

The sand bath sometimes produces an active perspiration. If this happens, interrupt the bath immediately and cover yourself again with dry sand, repeating this procedure 2 or 3 times, if necessary, to end perspiration.

Always finish the bath before arriving at a feeling of fatigue or cooling, which would be fatal. Keep in mind the length of this tolerance, and in subsequent baths increase only gradually. Begin with sessions from 10-15 minutes and increase them gradually to 1 or 2 hours, 2 or 3 times a day. Do not take them during digestive periods because they produce energy reactions.

Once out of the sand, dip completely in water; then cover yourself and rest before taking sun or renewing the bath.

Apart from sand baths, which can be local (and in this case rather longer), sand can be used in poultices—either for increasing the results of sand baths, or as a separate treatment for the same troubles and afflictions treated with sand baths. Heat the river or sea sand in an oven or frying pan. Put it into a bag which has been prepared beforehand and which is sufficiently large enough to cover the part to be treated. It should be about 1" thick. Apply it well heated and leave for 2-3 hours. Repeat as many times as necessary.

Techniques of sand baths have hardly changed over the centuries; the following text from the Greek Herodotus, reported by Dr. Hector Grasset, is more than two thousand years old:

"Sand treatment benefits those people suffering from asthma, pneumonia, gout, progressive paralysis, dropsy, and everyone who has chronic pain, because every ailing person, with the exception of small children, adapts himself to this treatment. Summer is the best season, choosing the most sunny days. In the morning, we prepare two or three graves of the same size as the patient, leaving them to be dried by sun heat. At home, the patient's food has to be well-distributed and he must previously have had good walks or other passive movements. When air heat is strong and sand sufficiently heated, the patient lies in the grave and is covered with as much sand as he can support. He must cover his head in order to avoid sunrays, placing over his eyes some protective object. Choose the best position for him; towards South at midday and during the first half of the day; towards North in the second half. Dry his face with a sponge soaked in cold water and if he suffers very much, also soak his mouth. If the patient feels that he does not heat himself or is cold due to sweat, he must say so; then the assistants should remove the sand which covers him, take him out of that grave, and place him again in a new one. If necessary, the change can be carried out once more in accordance with the illness and strength of the patient . . .

"We must bury in an inclined position those patients with asthma, pneumonia, stomach troubles those who have a bad appearance of anasarca hydropsy, and in a sitting position the hydropsical with ascites, and, if necessary, those who suffer from colon, liver, spleen, hip, gout or paralysis of feet or legs. At the end, we completely bury the patient because it is good for relaxation to spread throughout the whole body, and the useful effects of this treatment encompass the healthy parts also, especially with those who intend to take a cold bath immediately afterwards. Near the graves, it is necessary to have cabins of transparent material, pails of natural water and also bathing-suits, which are used by patients when they finish perspiring; after the bath, give them showers or massages with oil . . .

"With intermittent illnesses, the number of days of treatment are not less than 14 nor more than 21; but with hydropsicals, the number of days is in accordance with the remissions of the body's volume. If, after the 21st day of treatment, on arriving at a 'dead point' in its efficiency, it is advisable to take 2 or 3 days of rest and then renew the treatment again."

Mysterious Mud in Wyoming

The following stories were taken from a report written by Ray Pendergraft and distributed by a clay company in Wyoming.

"It lies up there near the top of the Big Horn Mountains in Wyoming. The deer and the elk come in the night and make tracks in it, as do many other animals, which is how it came to be discovered in the first place.

Emile Pascal, a trapper, was searching for likely spots to set his winter trap line, when he came onto an odd-looking cut bank composed of a whitish, cheese-like substance rising above a tiny lake where, to judge from the tracks, elk, deer, coyote and lynx seemed to congregate in large numbers.

So he made one of his "sets" there.

Two days later when he came to inspect his traps he noticed his hands, which had been badly chapped from the raw wind and snow, were coated with white cheesy mud; he looked at them and at the ice-bound lake and decided to wait until he got back to his cabin before washing them. When he did he found that they were not nearly as sore as they had been that morning; the cracks seemed to be healing and the skin softer. Perhaps the white mud had something to do with it.

The next time he made his rounds he brought back a

tobacco can of the stuff and tried it again. In a short time the chapping had disappeared.

The following summer Pascal filed on the outcropping a mineral claim and told his friends about the stuff. He let them try it. Soon reports of the strange stuff were circulating up and down the west slope of the Big Horns.

Carl Largent, a boy in Ten Sleep, had gotten a scratch on his thigh that wouldn't heal; it swelled up, turned red, and throbbed. The swelling continued, turned a greenish purple. So his dad took him to see a doctor over in Worland. The doctor began treatment, shaking his head; Carl's dad had waited too long.

The leg got worse. Till at last the doctor said: "I'm afraid that leg'll have to come off! It's gangrenous. If I had just gotten it sooner . . ."

But Carl's dad would not have it. "That leg stays on!"

He took the boy back to Ten Sleep. His friend, Pascal, had given him some funny-looking stuff, claiming it would heal sores. So now he mixed some with water till he had a thick paste, spread it generously all over the puffed-up leg, and bandaged it. After a while Carl dropped off to sleep. Some time in the night Carl's dad heard him calling. "Something's happened to my leg!"

His father came, unwrapped the bandage. The swelling was way down! Joyfully he applied a second poultice.

Today, years later, young Carl's leg is good as new—except for the scars.

Little Joan Monday, visiting at Grandma's in Worland one Thanksgiving Day, crawled onto the floor furnace before anyone could say, "Scat!" When she was yanked off screaming, both her tiny hands showed grill-shaped blisters.

Grandma had some of what they called the mountain stuff mixed up. She spread it over the child's palms in record time. Almost like magic Joan stopped screaming. Soon, both hands swathed in bandages, she was laughing again. There was no pain. The next day the blisters were gone, the grill marks barely visible. Joan did not even whimper when the red marks were touched.

Word of the stuff continued to spread locally. A rancher named Harvard had a son who had gotten himself stung by a swarm of bees; the stings poisoned him. Harvard used the stuff, and he swears, saved his boy's life. A member of a drilling crew got badly burned in an oil fire; the stuff, as they called it, was used. His burns healed quickly and with no complications."

The same report gives a few interesting insights about the amazing clay. Mr. Pendergraft quotes a doctor as saying, "We don't know what it is but it has something that does something to the bacteria. I feel it may be a natural antibiotic."

Mr. Pendergraft continues, "In view of this it is interesting to note a report issued by the United States Testing Company, Inc., of Hoboken, New Jersey. After noting that the clay is practically sterile, the report continued: 'The enclosed is a list of lab reports and case histories of work we have done on a mineral clay deposit that we feel should be further investigated, as we feel we've found something of interest to medical science.

'This deposit covers approximately seven hundred acres and its from five to ten feet thick and lies twelve to fifteen feet beneath ground surface; it is in a damp clay form when uncovered.

'Our own tests and case histories, though somewhat limited, have far exceeded our expectations.'

"Tests:

A dilution of ten to fifty CC of demineralized water gave the following results: A) inhibits growth of staph "A"; B) inhibits growth of Strep; C) inhibits growth of Sipplocci; D) inhibits growth of "E" Coli.

All tests were carried out under aseptic conditions incubated on blood over plates for forty-eight and seventy-two hours.

A solution using one gallon mineralized water and a two oz. scoop of dried pulverized clay applied to a wall of a room and cultures taken from all 4 walls shows a sterile culture of the coated wall for days; the other walls washed with plain water were contaminated each day.

Neutralized N 10 HCL one gram to one oz. more powder will turn the acid alkaline.

A patient taking 2 size 00 capsules of powder 4 times a day removed all symptoms of an active ulcer and hyperacidity in seven days.

A wet pack applied daily to a "boil" headed it out in three days and when it broke, a culture of the wound was sterile, the wound granulating from the inside out, in an additional forty-eight hours.

A 5 dieulitus ulcer, by spreading the dry powder on the ulcer and covering it each day, dried the ulcer in forty-eight hours and granulated it in 7 days.

A wet pack on corns and calluses of the toes and between the toes, left on three days, changed and left on an additional three days, will relieve all the symptoms and the corn just isn't there.

Used on allergic dermatitis in a reconstituted clay and washing the hands with soap made from the powder cleans up the dermatitis in seven to ten days.

A poultice on the body works as diathermy and greatly increases surface circulation.

Used as a poultice on the face and arms after having been burned from an explosion of coal-oil and wax, the pain was stopped almost immediately. Removed the dark coal-oil color from the burns and left them only a dark red; the area treated as above did not blister, the hands treated conventionally did blister. Treatment was a wet pack of the mineral three or four times a day.

Ring worm was cleared up by repeated applications of the solution.

Used on sore teats of milk cows it cleared up and toughened them much faster and better than available preparations.

As a facial pack it clears up pimples, leaving the skin smooth and soft.

Eczema treated by "everything" for ten years started clearing the hands up in two days; and in one week the hands were normal.

"Pink eye" was cleared up in a day and a half.

Used in powder form it cleared up "diaper rash" overnight.

Used in solution, it soothes and rests tired and sore eyes with no harmful effects.

With only the small facilities available to us, we have been unable to develop tests as completely as we would like, and as we feel the material justifies. We do not expect "miracles" but, there is something here that is doing something to bacteria and the body, to cause it to heal; we do not know what it is but feel it should be made available to more people.

We believe that there are possibilities for this as a staphylocide and possibly A.B.B. control and there is something here that gives relief almost immediately. We do have lab reports and documentary evidence of all our case histories."

"As part owner of the claim to the mine where the clay is abundant, I am convinced that its benefits should be widely known. Sooner or later this must happen."

Chapter 3
A FEW CASE HISTORIES

stomach ulcer

A public and eminent person had been suffering from a stomach ulcer for more than twenty years. He had been in and out of the hospital and was back in it a year ago. He was bleeding so badly that doctors felt he should undergo surgery. He was resting in his room when he suddenly remembered a friend who had assured him that clay would get him out of his troubles.

The sick person was in a New Jersey hospital 40 miles away from his friend. He immediately asked his wife to go to New York City and get some clay from the friend. The wife smuggled it into the hospital and gave it to her husband, who, after taking it three times, began to feel better. Two days later, he was out of the hospital, the following day he was back to work.

Another person, who had been suffering from an ulcer for the past ten years took the clay from toothpaste, for clay in powder form was not available then. After two days the pain vanished. However he took clay for another two weeks to make sure the pains would not return. Now everytime there is a recurrence on account of bad eating habits and social pressure he takes the clay, eats better, and the ulcer goes.

severe acne

A gentleman over thirty years old had suffered from this annoying disease for more than fifteen years. His problem was so severe that it looked more like abscesses than acne. It was all over his face even up to his head. He was so disfigured that not only could he not get a job but was ashamed to go out.

He started taking clay orally as well as in the form of masks, which he applied at night. He changed his diet of course and that helped to heal his sores very rapidly. After a month his face was all clear. Now you can tell by the condition of his face whether he ate healthy or bad foods. Anyway, he knows his cure and it takes him no more than a week or two to clear up slight recurrences due to exaggerated eating.

discal hernia

Mr. J. was suffering from sciatica so painful that he could barely get up. He consulted an acupuncturist and two osteopaths, who said surgery was necessary.

He decided to apply clay, two poultices a day, and one at night. He also took cold hip baths, lemon and clay orally and a recalcifying decoction. He did this for two months, very steadily.

By the third month, there was marked steady improvement and after this the condition became normal. Nevertheless he kept continuing the treatment at a slower pace for some time to ensure the cure.

double hernia

A man in his thirties was suffering from a double hernia in his abdomen; one eight years old and the other two years old. He was told that he should apply clay poultices on his abdomen before going to bed and leave them on overnight. He would take it off and apply another for the day time. After six to eight weeks, the eight year old hernia was completely healed and the two year old one was on its way to being healed.

infected ear

A three year old boy was suffering so much from an infection of the ear that a doctor advised the parents to immediately give antibiotics if they didn't want their son to have complications set in. The father refused to give antibiotics. He called a friend who knew about clay who advised him to apply two to three poultices a day on the back of the ear. After two days the pain was gone. They continued applying the poultices for an extra day or two to make sure that the infection was completely gone.

eye wound

In an accident, a patient's eye was struck by a well-handle thrown into the air. The cornea burst out, the iris was displaced and small crystal pieces from eye glasses aggravated the wound. Clay poultices were applied continually, renewed every hour. After the first day, the eye, which had appeared as a bloody paste, began to take on a better appearance. After three weeks, the cornea was rebuilt and the sight restored after three months. No surgical intervention was necessary.

stomach ulcer after two gastrectomies

In 1938 a priest aged 35 years was operated on for a stomach perforation produced by a pylorus ulcer, with a complication of peritonitis. Two years later, the ulcer reappeared with hemorrhages and greater pains, necessitating a second operation in 1942. Pain and hemorrhages again reappeared at the end of November 1952. Appetite diminished, strength declined, sleep became more difficult and more pain was felt. A third operation was foreseen.

At this time the patient became aware of clay treatment through reading the original French edition of Mr. Dextreit's work and decided to try it. Clay absorption began at the end of September, 1953. At the end of January, 1954, an improvement was felt, and by the end of February, pains disappeared, and the ulcer healed. Healing was complete and positive.

varicose ulcer

One patient, 72 years old, suffered very much from a varicose ulcer on her leg. After many doubts she decided to try applying clay poultices. The ulcer closed completely and the leg recovered normal appearance—much to the patient's astonishment as she had begun the treatment without any conviction and only because she was suffering so much that clay was a last resort.

dislocated vertebrae

Clay treatment succeeded in correcting dislocated cervical vertebrae of one patient. She can now turn her head from right to left easily and periodic trips to the doctor to put them in place are no longer necessary.

rheumatism of the hip

Thanks to clay, one patient was given an alternative to surgery of the hips, already envisaged by the rheumatologist. He was 37 at the first attack. The doctors could not understand that he could be struck with this arthrosis at his young age, but they did not propose any treatment. All he could do was wait while the disease took greater proportions and approached the stage of surgery. Then he heard of clay and other natural remedies. The clay poultices were applied every night.

Thirty months later, when he had not been suffering for a long time already, he returned for an X-ray. The results were such that the doctors, instead of becoming interested in his treatment, doubted the worth of the X-rays and all the previous examinations as well!

cataract

An 82 year old lady was resignedly waiting for her cataract to 'ripen' before undergoing surgery. Then she agreed to try application of clay poultices. It has been a year since it last bothered her. The improvement had been witnessed by her oculist.

birthmark

A birthmark on a patient's face was getting bigger. After putting clay on it for months, although quite irregularly, it almost disappeared, leaving only a light brown spot, like a beauty mark.

tonsillitis

One patient developed tonsillitis with high fever. The doctor that was called feared a serious inflammation and prescribed antibiotics. But instead of using them, he continued the clay poultices which he had already started. The third day the fever began to go down, the fifth day it was normal.

For precaution's sake, and to ensure the cure he continued taking clay-water and applying poultices on the liver for awhile.

dislocated collar bone

One woman writes that her son had his collar bone dislocated when he fell from his bicycle. Overnight clay poultices were applied every night for three months. The collar bone gradually came back to its normal place. She said afterwards, "I must confess that I was skeptical about getting the dislocated bones in place!"

amoebic dysentery

The nutritionist in her recent book *The Best of Linda Clark*, in the chapter "Have you tried clay?" related the following story:

"A friend of mine was afflicted with amoebic dysentery when she lived in a European country as a small child. Since nothing else helped, the doctors finally prescribed one teaspoon of regular, common tea, every hour, and nothing else. For a five year old child, this was a stringent treatment, but the doctors were trying to 'starve' the amoeba, they insisted. When the mother realized that they were also starving the child, she dismissed the doctors and took matters into her own hands. She spoon-fed moistened clay to her daughter and within a short time the amoeba had completely disappeared."

mononucleosis

A young man in his late twenties was told that he had mononucleosis and that he would have to rest a lot if he wanted to cure himself in a year or so. He took liquid clay orally for no more than a week and felt better. All the old users of clay were the most surprised when they were told the story.

fibrous tumor

A person of our acquaintance, after six months of repeated hemorrhages, was about to undergo surgery for the extraction of a fibrous tumor the size of an orange.

Approximately three weeks before the operation, she started application of clay on the lower abdomen. The operation was avoided; the tumor had gone down in the uterus and was evacuated through normal channels.

burns

A woman burned herself quite badly. It was taken care of in eight days by clay applications. Three poultices a day were applied—two during the day and one at night. There is now only a slight mark, even though the initial appearance of the burn was quite bad.

leg injury

One correspondent relates, "six months ago, a friend fell from his bicycle, wounding the front of his leg seriously. I immediately proposed clay poultices. The only answer he gave was a disbelieving stare.

Five months later he visited me again and his leg was in a very bad state. He had followed the standard treatment as was prescribed to him: pomades, cleansings. Seeing that finally he was really worried, I repeated my advice. He agreed, and I gave him clay on the spot (I always have some prepared). The best that could have happened, did. One and a half months later, everything was cured. There is only a bluish trace left, but no more pain."

breast cancer

A patient with cancer of the nipple had the nipple removed by surgery. After this, followed by radiation and radium applications, nodules appeared on the other nipple (a common occurrence—removing a cancerous growth is not at all curing cancer). An operation was foreseen with prospects of a limited life.

The patient changed to natural medicine, she modified her diet, took teas for the liver, and applied clay on the nodules and ganglions. Her state gradually improved. Unfortunately she then became the victim of an auto accident and had to be fitted with a plaster cast for a vertebral fracture. The surgeon agreed to open a window on the plaster to allow clay applications on the fractured area.

It is now more than ten years since this patient followed clay treatment and her present condition would appear enviable to many others.

ear cancer

There was a case of ear cancer in a patient 78 years old who had already been operated upon. The consultant specialists considered this relapse a forerunner to the unavoidable end; all medical or surgical treatment was considered a failure. The patient turned to clay.

Repeated applications of clay on the actual tumor produced the elimination of pus and black blood. Tissues began to be rebuilt after 8 months of treatment and the tumor closed almost entirely. Two years after his fatal condemnation (at the time of this report) the patient is still living, the trouble rapidly diminishing.

severe cut

A woman we know had a deep cut in the right thumb caused by a kitchen appliance. Clay poultices were applied immediately. The extensive bleeding of the wound stopped with the first applications. In the beginning the poultices were renewed as soon as the clay dried. After eight days the flesh was reconstituted and her finger was returned to normal.

crushed finger

A friend had her finger crushed by a door, but unfortunately did not think of clay until the next morning, after a bad night. After 48 hours the pain finally calmed down. Whenever the pain manifested itself, clay would soothe it.

After a few days, seeing her finger black and swollen, her daughter, who is a nurse, advised her to have it opened in a clinic, telling her that she would be given antibiotics. This woman preferred to continue with clay. Her nail fell off, but in a very short time her finger regained a normal appearance and the nail grew back.

severed finger

A 17-year old boy sliced his left index finger with a sickle. It was so deep that the finger was attached only by some flesh around the joint.

Twenty minutes later, without using a disinfectant, a clay poultice was applied and renewed frequently, day and night, for two days. Between the poultices a pellicle of onion (which is found between the layers), a natural antiseptic, allowed a dry bandage. From time to time the finger was exposed to air.

All the flesh then formed a crust of protection. In less than two weeks, everything was healed and even the traces disappeared.

Chapter 4
CLAY IN ANCIENT AND MODERN TIMES

The earth cure is as primitive and simple as it sounds. Modern times have established a stereotype of cure and treatment of disease which at first made it difficult for people to choose to heal themselves with simple natural means. It is good news that many people now realize that the earth itself is a healing source, along with all that grows on it. The following forms of cure from the living earth are known to be very effective in treating several kinds of diseases and for other purposes as well.

Clay Baths

The use of mud with high mineral content is very common at present in health resorts and clinics. This is a good idea, because its actions are powerful and helpful, although for maximum benefit it is necessary to complement them with a natural way of eating.

If it is not possible to go to these spas due to the inconvenience or expense, you can take advantage of the benefits of mud baths with a mixture of clay and water.

If you have a garden, dig a hole sufficiently long and deep enough in which to dip your whole body, once the hole has been filled with mud. To protect against cold, do this in the open air only during warm periods when the clay can be exposed to sunlight.

These baths can be taken inside in a trough, cask, etc., but never in a bath-tub as the clay would obstruct the drain-pipes. Mix the clay and water so as to obtain a clear paste. This bath can be used several times; each time add a little water, cold or hot, according to need.

Begin with daily baths of 5-10 minutes duration, then increase to 15-20 minutes. If they tire you, take them every second day or twice a week. After a month of treatment, rest for one month before resuming.

These baths are recommended for treatment of rheumatism and arthritis, osseous afflictions, for certain skin and blood illnesses and for certain kinds of paralysis.

Bathing specific parts of the body is equally possible, and is very effective; especially foot and hand baths in cases of rheumatism.

Slime Mud

This is the sandy clay deposits left by water on their withdrawal. Its properties are variable but definite. Ancient deposits of slime mud constitute the 'loess' (yellow earth), of which successive layers present different aspects. The inferior (lower) loess is virtually arable and predominantly chalky. It is the "argilette" of Normandy and the "terre douce" (sweet ground) of Picardy.

The upper level, reddish and rather sandy, is very rich in arable clay. It is the "terre a brique" (brick ground) of the districts of Paris.

All these grounds may be used when true clay is unavailable, but only for external use.

Clay Powdering

Finely ground clay is advisable for powdering babies, instead of talcum, which generally has medicinal substances but not clay activity. Don't hesitate to use clay powder on childish pimples or have them drink it, if necessary.

On ulcers, powdered clay performs an antiseptic action, favoring the rebuilding of harmed tissues. Powder sores, scars, inflammations, eczema, etc.

The use of very fine clay powder for a massage increases its efficiency.

Animals and Clay

A person who observes nature can witness the fact that animals instinctively use earth to cure themselves. Indeed, we owe much of our discovery in this field to animals. There is a sea resort in the Siberian forests of the Oussouri where the discovery of the curative properties of the earth was the result of observations of wounded animals, wild pigs, roe-deer, red deer and other animals who came to wallow in the benefactory mud. Dr. Em. Grommier has told the story of the elephant "Fil," who, with his kindred, purged himself with silicic-magnesic clay-marls and daubed himself with mud.

The French Army used it recently for veterinary purposes—when horses were afflicted with hoof gangrene, they were put in a stable, the floor of which had been dug up and kept wet so that the horses could kick in the mud. The animals went instinctively to the clay-mud where they found a remedy for their disease.

Animals seem to know instinctively the usefulness of contact with clay when they are ill or wounded. Those living wild do not hesitate to dip the affected area in mud. Domestic animals, too, turn to clay. A cat that is abscessed, wounded or ill will lie on a clay case (a large bin of clay covered with a cloth). Even when not ill, she will prefer this bed to one more comfortable.

Domestic and farm animals can be treated with clay. The method of treatment is the same as for human patients, the only difficulty being in the docility of the animal in accepting the treatment. Farm animals can be persuaded to dip themselves into a mud bath prepared by digging a large enough hole filled with clay and water. Cows have been cured of foot-and-mouth disease (apthous fever) with applications on the feet and daubs in the mouth. In certain countries, seriously ill animals are saved by daubing them completely with a mixture of clay and vinegar. Good results are also obtained by replacing vinegar with very salted water (sea salt).

For internal use, clay is also effective. It can be added to the drinking water (4 soupspoons per quart of unboiled water) and even mixed with food. It can be used in the fur —particularly for cats, who constantly lick their fur, thus absorbing it easily.

Agricultural Uses

Clay is able to replace all chemical fertilizers and can be used in the form of packs, daubings, cements, powders, etc.

Clay is the best pack for tree wounds. Make thick applications which will only stay on if the clay is solid enough. Once the clay has been put in place, it cannot be re-applied.

When transplanting or replanting, soak the roots of small plants in a clay bath and daub the roots of trees, bushes and big plants. For 5 quarts of mud add a coffee-cup full of a decoction of chamomile (1 oz. of flowers to 1 quart of water)—this is the maximum dose.

In acidic ground, recognized by the presence of daisies, moss or buttercups, clay can be added to improve the balance of the soil. When the soil is rather light (too sandy) prepare clay as if for a poultice, let it dry, grind, and spread it over the soil.

Added to organic debris, clay increases the production of humus and also the amount of carbon fixation in the soil.

Clay in Industry

Clay has many industrial uses. Many centuries before our era, the Chinese people used a certain kind of clay for decoloring greasy oils, according to M.C. Alexanian, Doctor of Physics. He adds that the Egyptians, Greeks and Romans clearly knew of this scouring and decoloring property. The frescoes of the 'fullonica' of Pompeii show the Roman bleachers trampling the cloths in clay-water—clay derives one of its names from this: "Fuller's earth."

Clay is still used today for decoloring oils, both mineral and vegetal—attapulgite, sepiolite, illite, etc. (5 grams of good clay being sufficient for decoloring 10^3 cm of a water solution to 0.1 of Methylene blue. It is also used for treating margarine, giving it the taste of butter). In the U.S. alone, 300,000 tons of "Fuller's earth" are used every year, of which 180,000 tons are used for treatment of oil-bearing products.

In North Africa, more than 100,000 tons of Bentonite are mined, mostly for the petroleum industry. Here clay, a natural silicate, is used as a catalyzer (it has remarkable resistance to being affected by chemicals) in the genesis of petroleum, determining a series of transformations of several organic materials. The essences of cracking are purified, passing under pressure over an absorbent clay. Thanks to clay, the 'catalytic cracking' allows the transformation of the gas-oil into a liquid burning essence, then into polymerizable gas, used in the manufacturing of synthetic rubber and other products. A white clay is used as a strengthening charge in the manufacture of natural rubber, for certain synthetic rubbers, thermoplastic material (such as vynilic resins), anti-acid paints, hydro-carbonated soaps.

Chapter 5
CLAY TREATMENTS

choosing clay

Clay may be obtained from herbalists and other merchants, as well as from quarries and the industries which use it in large quantities. In fact, it is good to always have some ready-made clay on hand, convenient for camping, car, etc. It is sold ready-made commercially (in health food and herbalist shops) in tubes. If clay is obtained from a ceramics supply outlet make sure that it is 'virgin' clay, that is, that it was extracted from the quarry without having undergone any treatment. Never use prepared clay baked or mixed with medicinal substances or any other additives.

There are many varieties of clay, and many different colors (green, red, yellow, grey, white, etc.). It is important to find the one most suited to the ailment or to the temperament of the patient. When we use nature's products we are not running to an inert substance, but to life. We must look until we find 'sympathy.'

Clay is alive. There are kindred links between clay and living beings, whether plant, animal or man. The same clay can produce a marvelous result in one person and seem 'inoperative' in another. Actually, it is always active, but only to a degree that is a function of the relationship between the person and the particular clay. When it seems inoperative, it is important to realize that it is that one particular clay which is not being very active, but not 'clay' in general. It would undoubtedly be possible to overcome this 'intolerance' by gradual habituation, but it is probably advisable to switch to a different clay. It may be necessary to get it from other districts or try many kinds in order to find the origin or color which is favorable. As a rule, clays obtained from the district you live in, act more in 'sympathy' than those from a far quarter, although there are exceptions. It would be best to try a few different kinds before determining which is the one for your specific needs.

Assuming that nothing in clay's composition explains its action on the organism, it will be necessary to refer to empirical evidence and opinions based on experience for guidance in selecting the most efficient variety of clay. In general, it seems that greenish clay is the most active. However, it is also the least tolerated in cases of hypersensitivity. Certainly it can be used initially, reserving the possibility of changing to another in the case of any disagreeable manifestations such as nervousness, cooling, etc.

before using

The more clay is exposed to sun, air and rainwater, the more active it will become. It allows clay to exercise its property of absorbing and storing a remarkable part of the energy of other elements, above all the sun. It is possible that its infinitesimally small particles constitute as many condensors capable of freeing withheld energy at the appeal of an opposite pole. Assuming the revitalizing action of clay, it may be possible to say it has the property of attracting the sun's magnetism upon initial exposure to light. It is this energy which it reconstitutes and gives out upon use. Perhaps it is this revitalizing action which accounts for its ability to fix the oxygen in water added to it.

The time for exposing clay to sunrays is just prior to an immediate need. For storing clay in its initial condition darkness is better; it can be kept indefinitely. It will grow no older in a dark container than it would have in the quarry from where it was taken.

At this point, it is necessary to add that even taken out and applied without an intermediary and long exposure to light, clay already possesses most of its wonderful properties. A graphic proof is that clay is quite irreplaceable for sustaining life in cavernous species that dwell in pitch-dark. These cave-dwellers, especially the Niphargus shrimps mentioned earlier, can only reproduce and develop themselves in clay. These animals would disappear and die if they were deprived of clay, although they are able to stand a lack of food for a long time.

two precautions

Clay does not adapt itself to the presence of other pharmaceutical medicines (even homeopathological ones); therefore, it is not advisable to combine its use with medical treatment. Sometimes patients under medical treatment are eager to know whether they can begin to use clay before finishing their treatment. It is not recommended, especially if used internally, as clay generally is inhibited by medicines. It is better for them to wait until ready to definitely and exclusively use the natural method of drinking clay. However, it is sometimes possible to combine external clay applications with medical treatment, especially for those people who still doubt clay's effectiveness.

As clay is so powerful, it is advisable to precede clay treatment with at least ten days of purifying teas and food (mostly raw fruit and vegetables; no meat, sugar, alcohol, or chemicals) in order to reduce the amount of harmful toxins in the body. In all cases, clay treatment should be accompanied by sensible and healthy eating habits.

internal use

The idea of clay taken orally is now accepted and does not produce unjustified feelings of revulsion as it did when it was unknown. This is in part due to the fact that its benefits are becoming better known, and also because it turns out to be not at all disagreeable to take. The visible evidence of the effectiveness of clay applied externally also inspires confidence in its internal use.

It is interesting to note that when mixed with water, clay does not granulate unless there is the unfortunate presence of sand. So, for drinking purposes it is best to choose a fine clay which does not crack in the teeth, one without sand. Use green clay from France. It is the type Raymond Dextreit uses and recommends. A few American nutritionists also find it to work best. It is available in most health food stores. The same clay could also be used for all sorts of other purposes such as skin problems, cuts, wounds etc.

measurements

The clay should be prepared, if possible, several hours or even a night in advance. Put a teaspoon of clay into half a glass of unboiled water. *Do not leave a metallic teaspoon in contact with clay.* It is best to drink clay in the morning after waking or at night on going to bed; however, even 15-20 minutes before eating is possible, although at least an hour would be better.

Clay modifies itself—its action changes according to the method of preparation (clay poured into water or vice versa, water onto dry clay, etc.) and according to the manner of drinking it or application. So it is possible to observe a tendency to 'obstruct' the bowels if drunk before breakfast, while quite a different effect may be manifested if it is taken in the evening. This action of the bowels is the normal and quick 'direct' effect but if we are looking for a sedation of stomach pains after eating, then we have to take the clay immediately before eating.

The first treatment of clay lasts three weeks, then after a rest of a week, treatment is renewed continuing during the following months at the rate of a week of treatment alternating with a week of rest.

Clay does remarkable work in restoring deficient organs and organic functions. It does not accomplish this by supplying the missing elements, but by aiding the organism to be able to fix and assimilate those elements where previously it was failing. These catalytic substances need only be present in infinitesimal doses. Therefore, it is unnecessary to absorb large quantities of clay; a teaspoon daily is a sufficient average.

We know that certain substances such as lycopodium, inoffensive and inoperative in large doses, becomes one of the most active medicines when taken in infinitesimal doses. Similarly, clay should be used in relatively small doses. *It is useless to take large doses because its action, as already said, is due to its radiations and not to quantities of particular elements.* It is not merely a pain-reliever; it must be used prudently especially when taken internally.

As has already been said, the average dose is a teaspoon for adults and half for children under 10 years, although in some bowel infections (tuberculosis, dysentery, etc.), the dose may be increased to two or three teaspoons a day.

When ingestion of clay is poorly tolerated, it is necessary to avoid injury by accustoming the organism to it slowly. Begin by drinking only the clayish water; introduce clay gradually until the daily dose of a teaspoon—the average per adult—is acceptable. Anyway, the absorbed quantity is only relatively important; there are people who, being unable to swallow clay and water, prefer to drink only the water after most of the clay has settled at the bottom of the glass, and they get satisfactory results.

If clay absorption produces nausea, mix it with a little water in order to form a kind of paste, make small balls like peas and let them dry. Swallow these instead of clay powder. For children, prepare this paste with some aromatic infusion (mint, eucalyptus, etc.) instead of water; and give the balls to suck as if they were caramels. People inclined to constipation can prepare the balls with a decoction of senna or rhubarb.

Babies will take a teaspoon of clayish water before three feedings every day.

In the case of rheumatism or sore throat, suck clay pieces or balls or simply take a teaspoon of powdered clay.

Sometimes clay sends forth a taste of petroleum, which does not alter its properties; quite the contrary, naphtha is a powerful antiseptic and clay is sometimes in contact with it in the ground.

As clay enriches the blood, it is advisable not to take too much when blood pressure is rather high—take only one or two small doses a day with water.

If clay causes constipation, dissolve it in a little more water and take it several times during the day, between meals. If the constipation presists, replace clay temporarily with a laxative tea.

This trouble can be eliminated by drinking a lot between meals so that the volume of liquid is sufficient to dilute three solid residues and evacuate them. In order to avoid this inconveniency—which is not all that common—in the beginning drink only the clayish water, leaving the sediment in the bottom of the glass.

Clay bricks are hardened and impermeabilized with an emulsion of a petroleum derivative. Thus, during clay treatment it may be prudent to restrain the use of domestic oils, whether or not this is really necessary. In fact this is a precautionary measure, because no incident has ever been reported involving the use of clay and the consumption of vegetable oil. In terms of experience only the consumption of mineral oil is to be mistrusted. On the other hand, it is advisable to drink a lot between meals (lemonade, teas, etc.).

All these precautions apply especially concerning afflictions in which clay is in direct contact through the digestive channel (stomach or duodenal ulcer, enteritis, etc.).

Clay for External Uses

Clay should not be prepared in a small bowl but in a deep bowl, wash-basin or a deep mixing bowl, or even in a large wooden trough, as with clay it is best to have a large amount. Use a container made of enamel, earthenware, porcelain, wood, or glass, but never of metal (aluminum, copper, iron) or plastic materials. For storing dry clay, plastic may not be unsuitable, especially considering that nowadays plastics are manufactured for every kind of food product and considered perfectly stable. However, for the mixture of clay and water it is advisable to use only those materials of recognized traditional stability.

Place clay inside, matching the surface distribution as much as possible. Keep a little dry clay nearby in case the mixture is too clear and has to be thickened; it is preferable for the mixture to be rather clear, as it is easier to thicken it by adding clay than to thin it by adding water. It is logical to prepare clay for several days use. For storing, just pour on a little water every day without touching the clay. If clay for poultices begins to harden before use, let it harden and when it is dry, grind it prior to a new preparation. Do not be afraid to prepare too much at one time. Prepared in advance, clay lays out for better homogeneity. You will observe that when well-prepared and regularly soaked in water, it is easier to use.

Add unboiled water to the clay in the container until it reaches a half inch or so over the clay—initially, it may take a few trials because all clays do not absorb the same percentage of water. Let the clay rest for some hours *without touching it*. When it is stirred up, it becomes sticky and difficult to handle. It loses its porosity becoming smooth and, in consequence, impermeable. Its possibilities of absorption are then very much reduced. It is not necessary to touch it before use; it dilutes itself alone quite well. Handle it as little as possible when placing it on the supporting cloth. Do not smooth its surface—it will settle naturally when put into place.

The prepared clay has to be a smooth, very homogeneous paste and not very concentrated—just enough to avoid falling apart. When possible, place the container in the sunshine, covering it with a gauze in order to avoid impurities.

clay temperature

Clay may be used cold, tepid or hot, depending on the specific problem. Each time it is used on a feverish or over-active or naturally warmed organ (e.g. lower-abdomen), it must be cold. A few minutes after applying the poultice, it should feel tepid. If the cold sensation persists, it is not advisable to continue the cold poultice. On the other hand, if the poultice starts to feel very hot, it is necessary to change it after 5 or 10 minutes. When clay is used for revitalization purposes, for osseous rebuilding, for kidneys, for gall bladder, liver, etc., it must be warm, or at least tepid.

The guiding principle is that 'every action is immediately followed by a reaction.' Thus, if we use the poultice on a feverish, angry or congested part, we have to refreshen it; but, if used with the goal of strengthening or revitalizing, we have to warm it. Applied on a weak or feeble organism or ogan, it is possible to make cold applications of cold water, air, or mud, but the overheating, which is the goal of this application, must follow rapidly.

For fever or congestion, where the cold treatment may be compared with the system of water circulation for cooling car engines, overheating is dangerous and must be avoided. In other cases, however, this cold treatment must bring about an overheating of the body due to the stimulation of organic functions such as oxidation and circulation. This means the body's temperature must rise slowly; *only when it produces this effect is the cold treatment beneficial.*

As with every rule, there are exceptions and there are weak or feeble people who will maintain poultices longer than necessary or remove them before the clay has had time to dry. In such cases as when the clay produces a disagreeable feeling of cooling or even when it does not warm on contact with flesh, it is advisable to place a bag of boiling water near the poultice or beside the patient's bed. There cannot be a good defense without heat.

In some cases clay may at first weaken the patient. This obstacle is not insurmountable and after a long or short period of adaptation, clay becomes more bearable. In fact, it is a phenomenon of revitalization that energy so developed produces an immediate, but temporary reaction, reflecting latent reserves. Do not force things; apply small poultices in several places until a favorable position is found where clay can be easily supported. Put regular poultices around these areas, gradually increasing the size and duration of their application, eventually reaching the desired zone of treatment.

It is interesting that a clay poultice can be active on a point far from the application site. It is not necessary for clay poultices to be in direct contact with the affected part, for clay acts on the whole body. In a dental crisis (an abscess or such), clay may be put in direct contact with the gum—but it has actually been proven more efficient to apply a large poultice on the cheek.

how to heat clay

It is necessary to avoid placing clay in direct contact with a powerful source of warmth. A double-boiler is the most convenient way that will still preserve all of the clay properties.

Place the container with the clay paste within another larger container filled with water to at least half the height of the clay container. Place everything on a fire and leave it there until the desired temperature is reached.

By placing it in the sunshine or by another source of mild warmth such as a radiator or a warm stove-top, it is possible in certain cases to sufficiently heat the clay.

If you have prepared enough clay in advance for several poultices, do not heat the entire poultice because clay cannot be warmed twice. In this case, place the poultice fully prepared on the covered lid of a pan of hot water.

A good method to induce natural heating of the poultice is to apply very hot wet compresses on the area of application in advance or simply use a bag of boiling water. The slight problem with heating the poultice initially is that this sometimes does not avoid cooling, but only prevents the patient from feeling the disagreeable sensation of cold clay in contact with the skin.

preparing the compress

Sometimes the use of a weaker clay compress is preferable to that of a poultice. To prepare it, it is necessary to make a clearer paste by combining less clay and more water than for a poultice. Just before using, stir it up in order to get a good mixture. It should adhere to a piece of cloth upon contact. Dip the piece of cloth into the clay, wring it out a little and place it on the part to be treated, using an intermediate cloth if necessary.

how to prepare a poultice

Place a piece of cloth folded in two or four parts on a table, bearing in mind that it has to be rather larger than the part to be treated.

With a palette-knife or a wooden spoon (neither metal or plastic material) spread an even layer of clay onto the prepared cloth. The thickness can vary from 1/4" to 1", according to need. Applying it as if it were an ointment will not get good results. Except when it is for a boil or similar treatment, clay can easily cover a surface of 4" × 8" with a thickness of 1" and often covers a surface of 8" × 12".

There are people who, for better handling of clay, prepare the poultices by mixing clay with wheat bran or flaxen flour in gauze. This is not correct, not only for reasons of comfort (as very dense clay is easy to handle) but also because the clay loses, at least partially, its beneficial properties. Besides, the traces which clay leaves are easily removed; even on an ulcer or open sore where clay must be placed directly onto flesh, if traces remain on removal of the first poultice, they are absorbed by the next one. When a gauze or cloth is placed between clay and skin, the poultice sometimes sticks less, allowing some air to come through, provoking the cooling of the poultice or produces a disagreeable feeling of diminishing the beneficial effects of the clay. For efficient action, it is necessary to place it directly onto the body. We can also help to obtain better contact by pressing the poultice into place, causing it to adhere well to the body.

This method has another important facet—that of helping to determine the duration of the application. Clay applied in direct contact can do this because, after producing its effects, it falls off as does ripe fruit off the tree. On an abscess boil, anthrax, etc., it takes about 20-30 minutes before the clay detaches itself, even when the poultice has been prepared with clay which is not so dense. When you notice that the clay has detached itself, its action has finished. It is not important to remove it immediately (especially if it is at night, it is not necessary to awaken to control the phenomenon of spontaneous detachment) but it is very important to bear in mind the minimum time of application.

Assuming normal activity, clay should be nearly dry on removal. In this case the poultice is easily withdrawn, leaving a minimum of clay stuck to the skin. If it does not detach easily, pour a little water between clay and skin. Rasp the remaining particles of clay on the skin and wash with cold or tepid water without soap. Never use alcohol or cologne water. Nevertheless, if clay has to be applied to a hairy or difficulty attainable part or if it has to be applied by a person who is treating himself alone, a piece of muslin, gauze or any other light cloth can be placed between the clay and the skin.

Once the poultice or compress is in place, cover it with a dry cloth, then fix it with:

—a bandage of light cloth, such as an 'ace' bandage.

—a small band of flannel or another warm fabric if the application is on kidneys, liver, abdomen or lungs.

—a sticky bandage if the area is not accessible for a simple bandage, or if it is very small.

—a 't' bandage if the application is perineal or rectal.

If the application is at the nape of the neck, bandage it to the forehead, not to the neck.

With regard to clay for external use, it is advisable to use a cabbage leaf instead of a cloth for covering clay placed on an inflamed organ, an abscess or another purulent sore. In these cases, clay dries very quickly; the cabbage-leaf slows this drying, as cabbage keeps fresh longer. This may also be put into practice for a large poultice to be kept overnight—otherwise, it would dry very rapidly (particularly with varicose ulcers).

rhythms of application

The duration and sequence of application depends on the case to be treated, the extent of the ailment, the temperament of the patient, his reactions to clay, the surface to be treated and all other variables.

The application can last from one hour to all night, according to the case. Thus, when treating a deep organ (liver, kidneys, stomach, etc.) we can leave the poultice for two hours as a minimum, sometimes three or four hours. They should be spaced well before and after meals. It must be remembered that these larger applications determine very important reactions and that the organism cannot withstand them for a very long time without the risk of weakness if they are renewed frequently, especially if the patient is continuing his normal pace of activity. One poultice a day is usually proper. Two poultices a day may be applied to a patient who is in bed or inactive, if he can withstand them without fatigue or excessive reactions.

If the application has the goal of revitalizing an organ, or rebuilding an osseous decalcified tissue (vertebrae, etc.) it may be left overnight, but it should be removed during the night, if it disturbs or if it becomes cold.

On the other hand, if treating an abscess or purulent ulcer for example, it is necessary to change the poultices every hour whenever possible, night and day, until the end or put cheese cloth between the clay and the skin (but an hour and a half. At night, apply compresses of clayish water renewing them once or twice. Finally, when tissues begin to be rebuilt, apply poultices every two hours with dry dressings during the night.

Clay is not a standard remedy to be applied indiscriminately disregarding specific considerations of the patient, his condition and the location and method of application. For a good result, it is necessary to individualize the methods of application and to make some trials prior to the application of a determined treatment.

The season, as well as the climate, can be of great importance in determining the temperature of the poultice; for instance, a cold poultice, well supported in summer or in a warm region, can become unbearable upon change of season or climate. A congested liver can present a good reaction to cold clay while a blocked-up gall bladder will generally need a hot application.

On the lower abdomen, where fermentation of improperly digested food occurs, leading to rises in temperature, cold poultices about 1" thick should be applied. Place clay in direct contact with the skin, or with a gauze in between on hairy areas. Poultices should be large. On the other hand, in certain afflictions, especially those of the bladder or ovaries, cold clay on the lower abdomen may be poorly tolerated, causing colic or other troubles. In such cases, tepid or even heated poultices must be applied.

With clay applications on the lower abdomen, as with the liver and especially with the stomach, it is necessary to apply them long after eating—essentially, completely out of the digestive period. Wait at least two hours after eating before applying a cold poultice; a hot one can be applied after one hour. Both must be removed at least one hour before eating in order to prevent clay reactions at the moment of beginning the first digestive phenomena. In general, the lower abdomen is where clay treatment must begin before any other application. However do not put clay on the abdomen during menstruation except if there is fever.

Clay succeeds by performing a powerful drainage action and attracts all the substances of negative radiation. It is perfectly understandable then that all the toxins of the body will direct themselves towards the treated part when clay is applied. Therefore, it is possible and even probable that on beginning the treatment a flaring up of the ailment will be produced; this is only an apparent and not a real worsening; it is due to the cleansing of the ulcer or treated part.

can clay provoke reactions?

With every natural remedy helping either to directly rebuild the organism, or to liberate and eliminate those substances which harm it, it is always possible that there will be disagreeable reactions. For example, a varicose ulcer will at first enlarge itself, the dead flesh of the periphery will fall off, the surface inflate and pus or blood can appear. Pain may even increase for some time but it will decrease later and finally disappear with a definite closing of the ulcer and rebuilding of healthy tissues.

This is why it is advised before beginning a natural treatment to be sufficiently informed of its possibilities and its development. When a reaction is foreseen, it is more easily controlled. We must not be afraid of these reactions; on the contrary, they are desirable, for they are a sign that the organism is responding to this intervention.

Of course violent reactions are never desired; do not

hesitate to temper too strong a reaction. Replace the clay poultice for another of wheat bran and ivy leaves if pain is very violent. Remove the clay poultice if it is the origin of disagreeable manifestations (nervousness, itching, burning sensations, cooling, etc.). When the disturbance is gone, recommence to whatever extent can be tolerated. More frequently, though, clay will act quite the contrary by calming intense pains.

Because the first action of clay is to drain abnormal particles towards the treated part and to cleanse ulcers, sometimes its immediate effect is to extend the ulcer, as mentioned above. In case of internal ulcers, as in any deep cancer (stomach, uterus, etc.) it is necessary to avoid such an extension that could touch essential neighboring organs or drive the vital reserves of the patient to exhaustion. Therefore, it might be best to begin with a mild action, applying a very small, thin poultice (less than ½"). After a few days, increase the size of the poultices, and after that the thickness may be increased. Arrive gradually at a poultice measuring about 8-12" long, 6-8" wide and ¾-1" thick. Don't increase both size and thickness simultaneously, but in accordance with the tolerance of previous applications that were without trouble, disorders or adverse reaction.

It is also advisable to precede the treatment with laxative teas, a fruit or lemon treatment, vegetarian nourishment and the absorption of clay by oral route, in order to greatly reduce the amount of toxins in the organism. It is only after ten days of this preparation that clay treatment should begin.

Once begun, do not interrupt a clay treatment, not even provisionally (presuming there are no adverse reactions). Clay is a very active agent; its application produces phenomena which start a chain reaction in the whole organism; to disturb the reaction once it has been started is hazardous. Just as it is useless to start a train and then suddenly stop it—it must reach its destination. Here, the terminal is good health.

Since the clay has a very powerful action (in the reactions it produces and the energy it frees) do not apply it on two different places at the same time. If, for example, a poultice is applied on the lower abdomen, it is advisable to wait one hour or more after it is removed before applying another on any different organ. This waiting period may be reduced to 30 minutes or less in certain cases.

In principle a clay application must not produce trouble or a sensation of pain. If, for example, a poultice placed on an abscess or boil dries it in half an hour, take it off without waiting the hour. If on the spinal column the poultice produces a cool feeling, even when applied hot, then take it off immediately and do not leave it overnight. When the application is made on a feverish or overheated part, it is necessary to take it out before the clay becomes warm; while if the goal is revitalization, that is to say, overheating, it is necessary to take it off before the clay cools.

Sometimes an obstacle arises in clay treatment which can hinder its continuation: the appearance of red patches or eruptions accompanied by unbearable itching. The explanation is that perhaps acid substances flowing from internal regions pass through the tissues attracted by clay. The fact that this itching stops after clay applications would confirm this hypothesis.

There may be other phenomena but they have no importance if the treatment can continue. Try to diminish these eruptions and appease the itching by applying a soupspoon of tepid water stirred progressively into clay to pomade density, and applied after the poultice. Protect clothes and bed sheets with a cloth. If the poultice has been applied in the evening and left all night, this ointment should be applied in the morning.

The following evening try to apply the poultice again; in the case of disagreeable phenomena, several continued evenings. Recommence the clay application when everything is normal. In addition, drink an herbal tea. Even at the end of treatment, do not stop the clay applications suddenly but lessen them gradually (every day, then twice a week, etc.). It is necessary to continue the applications more or less intensively to the last disappearance of the problem, until even the smallest piece of new skin over scars has properly grown in. Do not stop until the process is completely finished.

after use

Throw clay away after use, because it will be devitalized and impregnated with the toxins it absorbs. Whether it has been used on an ulcer or not, it is not able to be used again and is best thrown into a place where it cannot be touched. Wash the cloths which can be used again when dry.

It is possible to speculate that, exposed again to the elements and to its natural 'nourishment,' clay will recover from its overcharges and regain the greatest part of its potentialities. This has yet to be tested and proven. Anyway, it is certain the clay would need a long rest period. Nor is buying price all that high so as to inhibit the replacement of used clay.

When clay is needed for lengthy and difficult treatment look for a source of cheap clay such as in a quarry, brick factory, or a ceramic plant. Of course, handling this clay, generally in big damp blocks, is not very convenient.

Chapter 6
CLAY CURES
FOR MODERN AILMENTS

This portion of the book is not intended to be a complete guide to clay cures.* All the different types of diseases are not mentioned here, for the simple reason that clay is not known to have been used for some diseases, at least we do not have strong evidence that it was used with some of them. Clay may work for diseases other than the ones mentioned here, whether it is known by some people or not. The fact is that since clay, being the polyvalent healing agent that it is known to be, is especially a blood purifier, it would not be surprising to learn of other wonders it might accomplish.

This leaves the reader with the option and freedom to try clay wherever he thinks it would help. This does not mean that he should go so far as to experiment with it everywhere without having given the new matter any thought. He should at first refer to several sourcebooks which discuss many different diseases and their symptoms to find out if there is any corresponding case, in terms of symptoms or any other similarities. This would be a starting point for him. In addition, once he has decided to start the clay cure, he should not go full force with it at first; he should start with short periods of use whether

*For this, read *Our Earth, Our Care* by Michel Abehsera.

he drinks the clay or applies it as a poultice. For example, when taken orally, clay should be used with care by people who suffer from hypertension. It is so rich that it raises the tension of those who have the disease. In this particular case they should be careful not to use too much; rather only the liquid that was mixed with the clay should be taken.

The text for every disease was made succinct to keep the book small and handy. If the reader wishes to have more details on one particular disease, he should consult *Our Earth, Our Cure*, by Michel Abehsera. This book is especially good for those who also desire to acquaint themselves with vegetarianism.

The reader should be made aware of the fact that the cures for the diseases that are described here are not obtained by using clay alone. In these particular cases clay helps a great deal. The reader should consult books on healing, preferably of a vegetarian nature, for his own sake; in this manner he will ensure for himself a complete cure.

May you use good judgment for your own physical being and perhaps others. Good health, then . . .

abscesses and boils

The treatment has to include the draining of the liver with appropriate plants. The intestines, kidneys and bladder also have to undergo cleansing.

Every morning take liquid clay on an empty stomach.

Before lunch have an herbal preparation good for the liver, and before dinner take any food or herb tea which is good for blood purification. Take hot water mixed with lemon after dinner (half a lemon squeezed in a glass of water).

Put a poultice of clay on the liver before going to bed.

Be careful not to touch the affected area, for this would retard the healing which depends so much on cleansing and purifying.

Apply clay poultices on the affected area, renewing them every hour, more or less, depending on the condition. The clay should be prepared soft for it dries very quickly. Clay poultices are perhaps the most active of all auxiliaries; they are best in helping pus eliminate through the outlet of the infection. Apply the clay until there are shooting pains. Then temporarily interrupt the clay treatment and use one of the following: a poultice of cooked onion, or a plaster prepared by diluting 1-2 teaspons of sea salt in some water and placing it on a flame, stirring constantly. Add clay powder until it becomes a heavy batter. Continue to stir for awhile and remove from fire. Place on a thin cloth and apply this very hot against the skin. Put one plaster on at night and one in the morning. Keep in place permanently. Cabbage leaves may also be alternated with the clay poultices; cook whole leaves in a mixture of equal parts of lemon juice and water for several hours and apply.

Once the abscess has 'ripened,' meaning the pus is gathered under the skin, resume the regular clay poultices in the daytime. At night, use a large wet compress (cheese cloth soaked in clayish water). Do not cover with anything that does not allow it to breathe; rather, cover with a cabbage leaf which will maintain the humidity and let air enter. Place a cheese cloth on top of the cabbage.

Keep the area humid, so that the cavity does not close, keeping non-evacuated matters inside.

By prolonging the clay applications even when the abscess or boil is well-emptied, the chances of a scar remaining are considerably reduced. Space the poultices further apart and leave them on for 2-4 hours. Between poultices wash the area with unboiled salt water (1 handful of salt in 1 quart of water).

acne

People like to believe that acne is a juvenile problem, and yet people of all ages suffer from it. Among older people acne comes in different forms: a variety of crusty seborrhoea is manifested by yellow or gray crusts appearing on the nose and cheeks. In all cases of acne, the primary step is to bring the intestinal functions to normal. Either the evacuations are insufficient or the feces lack consistency or color, or else they are too colored.

Half a glass of liquid clay every morning on an empty stomach will get rid of a great part of the toxic products.

Stimulate the liver with a mixture of olive oil and lemon juice (one teaspoon of each, mixed) in the morning. Alternate this with the liquid clay weekly.

Eat only fruits, vegetables (often raw), cereals, dried fruits, yogurt, buttermilk and fresh eggs (soft-boiled). Use honey instead of sugar, very sparingly.

allergies

The organism is full of toxins. There is no other way to permanently cure an allergy other than by getting rid of these toxins. For this take half a glass of liquid clay every morning. Clay poultices on the liver before going to bed will help greatly.

Drink water and lemon juice mixture (half a lemon squeezed in a glass of hot water) twice a day. Apple cider vinegar* and water is also good.

alkalosis

An acute acid condition can often lead to alkalosis which is altogether different from the slightly alkaline pH of a healthy and normal person.

A person who follows a healthy and balanced diet has a blood on the alkaline side. This is what keeps him from contracting most bad diseases.

Alkalosis is a pathological state of over-alkalinity in which the healthy exhange of potassium and sodium does not take place. An organism which suffers from alkalosis is dangerously susceptible to disease because the nerves, muscles and organs are not in a normal active condition to prevent the spreading of the disease. Normal potassium and sodium exchanges keep the organism on the alert, letting nothing serious happen.

Besides beginning a good diet of vegetables, fruits and cereals (buckwheat, brown rice, rye, millet) take liquid clay once a day, preferably in the morning. Half a lemon squeezed in a cup of hot water twice a day is also good.

*We have found Sterling brand to be the best.

anemia

Knowing that blood passes through the liver, where it is purified and completed, and where it receives most of the nutritive elements, and knowing that the liver produces a factor of maturation of the red blood cells and regularizes their iron content, it is easy to conceive how anemia takes place.

It is vain to fight anemia with calf-liver for it introduces a large number of dangerous products which work against the process of assimilation.

A great error made is that of looking for the strongest types of food containing reconstituents and trying to absorb as much of them as possible.

When blood is anemic, this means the whole organism is deficient. It is proper, then, to introduce change without shocks. In this case too strong a type of food can worsen the situation.

Take liquid clay every morning on an empty stomach.

Eat plenty of green vegetables and grains.

Also take any herb preparation that aids the digestive process.

arthritis

Arthritis is mostly an inflammatory affliction of the joints. The synovial lesions reach the cartilages, then the bones, which eventually end up in deformation or ankylosis.

This disease comes principally from a predominance of acidic wastes in the blood which is caused by the transformation of nitrogenous excesses coming from food which become acid, and also by the acidic residues of the muscular activity. To this add acids coming directly from food, alcohol and coffee.

The most urgent thing to do is to begin a good diet which excludes all the harmful acidic foods—no starches, sugar, white bread, meats, etc. Take herb teas to cleanse the liver and the kidneys.

Apply clay poultices on the places that are mostly affected. Leave them in place several hours. They are very efficient. It is often better to apply them before going to bed and leave them overnight.

arthritis of the gums

Gum arthritis causes the teeth first to loosen and then fall out for there is no more support for them. Due to this loosening, food particles get in between the root and the gums and cause inflammation and putrefaction of harmful germs.

It is very rare to save the very loosened teeth; however, before having them pulled some strict measures should be tried.

Use clay toothpaste. Afterwards wash the mouth either with salted water or a mixture of water and lemon. Use a medium hard toothbrush. Brush vigorously in a vertical movement. (Never brush horizontally across the teeth.) Do not worry if any bleeding occurs. Brush the gums, not the teeth, always starting from the base of the gum.

After the brushing, massage the gums with the thumbs, the upper gums in a downward movement and the lower gums in an upward movement. The purpose of this massage is to put back the flesh on the gums, to get rid of the food particles that are stuck between the gum and the root, and to firm the tissues. Massage this way two or three times a day (using water-lemon mixture or salted water) depending on the condition. In addition to the massages, add mouth baths with salted water (sea salt, 1 teaspoon in a glass of water).

Suck on a piece of clay before going to bed.

bruises, bumps and blows

We should not neglect any discolorations or swellings, as some ligaments or vessels may be broken, or some nerves injured.

For healing the congestive state, it is necessary to apply cold clay poultices from 1/2-1 inch thick. Leave on for 2 hours, or less if the clay heats or dries rapidly.

There is no danger in continuing to apply poultices. The more are applied, the faster will be the healing. It is necessary to continue the applications until total disappearance of pain.

Every night, use a compress of clayish water and leave overnight.

burns

Burns treated with clay heal better, more rapidly and leave less traces than other methods, especially if the clay is applied immediately.

Apply cold clay, in thick poultices, with gauze between the clay and the sore. After one hour, remove the poultice, leaving the gauze if it has adhered. In cases of deep and extended burns when rags or cloth have adhered to the wound, leave them and apply the clay as previously indicated. The clay should have several points of contact with the burn, though.

Clay eliminates all risks of infection and absorbs all the impurities and foreign bodies apt to be found in the burn. It also eliminates the destroyed cells, enabling cellular rebuilding.

Renew the application day and night, changing them every hour, until the appearance of new tissues. Then reduce the frequency of application, but not to less than 3 or 4 poultices a day, and leave the poultices in place for two hours each, until the tissues are virtually rebuilt.

If the burns are on the feet or hands dip them directly into a container of clay paste. It is necessary to remain immersed for an hour so that no trace of the burn will remain on completion of this mud bath. For extended burns, it is advisable to dip the whole body into a large container of clay. Do not forget all other measures for maintaining a general healthy state.

ear infection

It is better not to eat in this case, even if the fever is not high. Drink a lot to cleanse the viscera. Take laxatives and diuretics; liquid clay every morning on an empty stomach; water and lemon mixture (up to one whole lemon in a glass of hot water); thyme infusions, etc.

Apply clay poultices 1 inch thick on the nape of the. neck. These poultices should cover the whole area of the nape of the neck, from one ear to the other. Dextreit even recommends that it should cover the ears themselves in which case place a piece of cotton in each ear to protect it.

Apply clay poultices on the lower abdomen 3-4 times a day, each one lasting 2-3 hours. Cold hip baths are excellent for activating the circulation. They should last no more than 2-5 minutes.

A few drops of lemon juice will also greatly help. Put a few drops in the ear and then a piece of cotton.

If possible take nose baths in liquid clay. Plunge the nose in the solution; close one nostril and breathe in with the free one. Do the same with the other nostril. Do this a few times, once a day.

eczema

Treating eczema exclusively with skin medication leads to a worsening of the internal condition. A good diet must be taken along with specific herb teas good for the liver.

With the oozing eczema the surface of the skin is red and humid; it dries up, forming small crusts which flake off when others are formed.

The dry eczema is red and shiny. The skin is constantly renewed through peeling.

Take liquid clay in the morning for a week and olive

oil-lemon (one teaspoon mixed with the juice of a lemon) the following week. Promote good circulation with short cold hip baths.

Apply thick clay poultices on the liver and lower abdomen in the evening, one day on one organ, the next on the other, and so on. Bandage and leave overnight.

For local treatment one should experiment with different preparations. In general, the dry eczema is treated with a mixture of olive oil and clay (2 tablespoons of oil, 1 of water and 1 of clay powder. Mix well). Coat the affected part and bandage.

The oozing eczema is treated by simply powdering it with clay. However, in case of inflammation, use a thick, broad clay poultice and keep in place for approximately two hours.

Chapped eczema should be given special lotions and local baths in an infusion of wild geranium (wild alum root) and absinth: a heaping tablespoon of each in a quart of boiling water. This preparation cleans the skin and activates peeling. In certain cases, both the baths and the mixture of clay-oil may be used.

If the eczema is infected, put a handful of box-tree leaves in a quart of water; bring to a boil and simmer 10-15 minutes. Alternate it with the clay poultice.

When the eruptions are accompanied by burning sensations, swelling and other discomforts, apply hot poultices of a mixture of elder-tree flowers (4, 6 or 8 tablespoons and enough whole wheat flour to make a paste when the water is added). Cook the mixture in a small amount of water for a few minutes. Place on a cheese cloth and apply hot.

These local treatments will help a lot. However, a true

and complete cure can be obtained only in combination with treatment of the fundamental problem.

fibrous tumors in the uterus

As for almost every disease this one cannot be taken care of with only symptomatic treatment. No toxic foods of any sort should be given. A good healthy diet should be eaten.

Lemon is good for accelerating the elimination of substances in excess and for contributing to the fixation of useful elements. Take 2-6 lemons a day, depending on tolerance.

Clay is an amazing remedy for fibrous tumors. It should be taken orally for the same reasons as the lemon. Take ½ glass of liquid clay once a day on an empty stomach.

Used externally, clay accomplishes wonders when accompanied by natural medicine and food.

Dextreit tells of a woman with a fibrous tumor in her uterus which caused serious hemorrhages during menstruation which was treated with clay. She drank it and applied poultices on her lower abdomen. After 3 months of treatment, an examination in a hospital produced this conclusion: "uterus is in the condition of a person of twenty." The patient was 50 years old.

In another case of an ovarian cyst, even specialists feared the operation which seemed unavoidable. However, four months of clay applications resulted in a significant reduction of the cyst (at first to the size of an ostrich egg—it had been much larger), making it possible to avoid the operation. Applications of poultices continued until the total disappearance of the cyst.

Spectacular results were often registered after a few weeks of treatment; however, it should be made clear that usually it takes months and sometimes even years, (in the case of fibrous tumors that do not bleed) to get rid of it completely.

For the first two months apply a poultice a day on the lower abdomen, interrupting it only at the period of menstruation.

The poultice must remain in place at least 2 hours. It can remain overnight if applied just before going to bed, unless it is too bothersome. The poultice must be approximately 10-12 inches large and 1 inch thick. The clay must be well against the skin (put a cheese cloth on hairy areas only). Begin first with cold clay; only if it is not tolerated should it be warmed up slightly.

In cases of heavy losses of blood prepare a decoction of oak bark. Use 4 oz. per quart. Boil 10-15 minutes and use as a very slow douche.

flat feet

Attempting to remedy this abnormality with orthopedic methods may be an error with dangerous consequences.

A good healthy way of eating should be followed. Infusions of plants should be given, especially those good for the liver such as thyme, rosemary, artichoke, dandelion, asparagus, shepherd's purse.

Every morning make a friction (light massage) of the

whole foot with a mixture of camphor oil and grated garlic (2:1). At night place a 1-inch thick poultice on the whole foot. The clay should heat up a bit; if it does not, heat it up to room temperature before applying. This can be done either on a radiator or in a double boiler.

fractures

The use of clay, rather than plaster casts, is recommended. It allows for faster results and eliminates the complications which might result from the use of plaster.

Plaster has only a passive action—that of immobilizing the parts to be rejoined. Clay is an active agent; with its vitalizing radiation and absorbent power, it participates effectively in the repair of the fracture.

First fix the bone in place with splints, although if the parts are displaced, as in a compound fracture, a specialist should be called. If a cast is unavoidable, ask the specialist if it is possible to leave some 'windows' through which clay may be applied.

Apply a uniform layer 1 inch thick, cold or slightly lukewarm. If there is a sore, change the clay every 2 hours. Otherwise, twice a week will suffice. Shave the hair or put cheese cloth between the clay and the skin (but direct contact is always preferable). Wash the skin with plain water (no soap or alcohol), between the poultices.

headaches

Headaches often come from bad digestion and fermentations in the intestines. A hot foot bath with either a decoction of red-grape vine leaves or mustard flour will greatly alleviate the pain. Apply clay on the forehead using $1/2$-inch thick poultices which are kept in place 1-$1^1/2$ hours.

In case of persistent headaches, apply 1-inch thick poultices on the nape of the neck which are kept on for 1 hour, alternating these with the former, once on the forehead, once on the nape of the neck.

Headaches will always come back unless the eating habits are changed. Most of the time the most violent headaches will disappear with an enema.

hemorrhages

Cold is the best treatment for hemorrhage. Thus apply clay poultices or simply cold compresses on the parts that are closest to the spot where the bleeding occurs.

In cases of uterine hemorrhage, apply clay on the abdomen every 2-3 hours, several times. To stop nosebleeding, apply the clay on the nape of the neck; also breathe in lemon juice.

For eye hemorrhages apply clay on the eye. Make poultices less than $1/2$-inch thick and place gauze in between, until the bleeding stops.

Whenever hemorrhages occur, use thick poultices, large enough to well overlap the wound.

Use lemon juice or salted water (sea salt) as a disinfectant.

hernia

Possibilities of healing depend on the age of the hernia. According to Dextreit a total healing of a hernia one or two years old is almost certain, but for one older than that, we can only hope for a complete cure.

The first element of treatment is the bandage for supporting clay poultices; it is necessary to make it solid in order to maintain support for some months of use.

Apply cold poultices, more than $1/2$-inch thick and somewhat larger than the affected part. Bandage in place for 2-4 hours. If it is not possible to change poultices every four hours, at least remove it and replace it with a cotton pad (prepared in advance) the same volume as the poultice. *Do not heave the hernia without support until it is completely reabsorbed..*

Morning and evening, lightly massage the treated part with a mixture of olive oil and chopped garlic. This massage must be carried out by another person, because the patient must be lying down.

Do not make any effort or movement when the bandage is not in place. As the hernia is being absorbed, the use of poultices and pad should be gradually diminished until the final disappearance of the hernia.

lumbago

The person suffering from a lumbago finds it necessary to lie down, remaining motionless. The return to normal condition may take time, for the torn ligaments must heal. It would be wise to use clay applications as long as possible for it may be that the lumbago is caused by a compressing of the disc which is placed between the 4th and 5th lumbar vertebrae or by chronic rheumatism of the spine.

Besides clay it would be helpful to massage the area with camphor oil and grated garlic (the oil should be as hot as bearable). Use two parts of oil to one part of grated garlic. Apply on the skin a bit at a time and massage until the oil is absorbed by the skin. Repeat the operation a few times, heating the oil if necessary.

lymphatitis

This inflammation of the lymphatic vessels is treated as for abscesses and carbuncles, as far as the general treatment of the organism is concerned. Treat the inflamed area with repeated applications of clay poultices, left on for 2-4 hours.

mumps

This inflammation of the salivary and parotid glands may affect the testicles, ovaries, mammary glands, pancreas and thyroid.

Follow a vegetarian diet. Eat small amounts of food. Take liquid clay every morning on an empty stomach and herbal teas such as sage, rosemary and thyme.

The child must remain in bed only if there is fever. In such a case, he should get up only to take cold hip baths 2-4 times a day depending on the severity of the temperature. Avoid solid food when there is temperature.

Apply clay poultices 1/2-inch thick, 3-4 times a day on the salivary and parotid glands, alternating with the genital organs. Keep each one on for 2 hours.

To prevent possible meningitis, apply a 'helmet' of cabbage leaves (3-4 layers) on the head, bandaging it in place. It should be replaced after 8 hours.

painful menstruation

If major troubles occur—if the menstruation is very abundant, insufficient, too painful or accompanied by several clots, mucosities or skin, apply a clay poultice on the lower abdomen every night before going to bed, which should be kept on overnight unless it causes discomfort. For minor troubles it is sometimes sufficient to apply these poultices only for 10 days preceding menstruation. Interrupt the application during the menstrual period, after that, resume applying them.

The applications can be continued even if the menstruation takes the form of hemorrhage; *be sure to slightly warm up the poultices in order not to create a congestive state.* According to Dextreit one of the best treatments for hemorrhage consists of applying fresh climbing ivy leaves on the top of the poultice, the stems against the clay. Renew the poultices every 2-3 hours during the day and every time the clay becomes warm during the night.

Of course a good diet must absolutely be eaten. Also take plants such as marigold and nasturtium which are rich in female hormones. Make infusions and drink 2-3 times a day. Sage is one of the best for this purpose.

psoriasis

Dextreit writes that most people cure this to a certain extent by exposing themselves to the sun. However, some people experience an aggravation of the symptoms by doing so. Those who were never able to tolerate sunbathing and ocean swimming will probably not find relief in this practice.

Those for whom being near the ocean is favorable should know that only by coming back to it for 2 or 3 consecutive years can they hope for a lasting cure. In the meantime they should pay close attention to their way of eating.

shingles

Use clay poultices immediately after the appearance of the blisters and feelings of pain. There is no reason to hesitate; even if it is the wrong diagnosis, there is no risk with clay —it only helps.

At the beginning of the treatment, renew the poultices every 2 or 3 hours. Later on, when the eruptions and the pain lessen, reduce the number until they are being applied only once or twice in a 24 hour period. Do not stop the poultices abruptly, continue for a few weeks to make sure that everything has been eliminated.

spine problem

Raymond Dextreit writes the following: "We have personally supervised enough natural treatments of various afflictions of the spine to be in a position to state that there are very few people who cannot find a solution to their trouble. Many people who were condemned to an orthopedic corset, bone surgery or immobilization have now been able to resume normal activities after a few months of natural treatment."

Food should be varied. Eat plenty of vegetables. It has been found that in all bone afflictions there is revealed a deficiency of silica, which is found in the outer layer of vegetables in general and cereals in particular.* Avoid all kinds of acidifying food, for they are responsible for weakening bone structure. Mixtures of food are great acidifying agents. Lemon, however, which may be acid, is not an acidifying food especially when taken in proper quantity and time. It should not be eaten with the meals, especially with such foods as grains, breads and starches.

Every day certain movements which aim at moving the vertebrae in all directions should be done. Walking, biking, gardening, etc. are excellent exercises which help

---

*an organic extract of silica, taken from the horsetail plant (richest in silica), is available at health food stores.

strengthen the spine. They should be done gently of course and one should not prolong them more than necessary.

According to Dextreit, the most efficient of all remedies is clay. Although some afflictions necessitate a longer treatment, six months of daily applications will usually take very good care of the most tenacious afflictions.

Dextreit relates the case of a boy 11 years old with cervical adenitis and decalcification of the vertebral column. Clay poultices were applied on the spleen and ganglions and the boy also took clay orally. First one ganglion burst then another, and his general state improved as well. The treatment had begun at the end of October and the parents considered the boy quite healed the following spring.

In most cases it would suffice to apply clay each night before going to bed; the poultice should be 3/4-1 inch thick, 6-8 inches wide and left on overnight. If clay is not tolerated cold, which is best, apply it slightly lukewarm, heating it with steam in a double boiler. It should be removed immediately if it causes any feeling of cold inside the body.

Clay should be prepared in such a manner as to remain flexible and conform to the body. It should be compact, neither too liquid nor too dry.

If two different places need treatment (for example in case of a double scoliosis, or a cyphosis associated with a lordosis), alternate the applications, one evening on one place, and the next on the other.

A massage of a mixture of two parts camphor oil to one part chopped garlic should be given every night. Proceed from the base of the spine upward, using a clockwise movement which starts at a point on the spine itself and extends out a few inches. This can last 10-15 minutes.

The back of the person receiving the massage should be maintained curved. Place a thick pillow under his abdomen in order for the penetration to be more efficient. After the massage apply the clay, being careful to remove all traces of remaining oil.

sprains

The most simple and efficient way to treat a sprain is to first place the injured part under a thin stream of cold water for 20-30 minutes.

Then apply thick poultices of clay that should be left in place for 3-4 hours. The one applied before going to bed can remain in place overnight.

Hot baths with salted water help ease pain. After the first day, take one every day for 15-20 minutes. After 2 or 3 days of clay applications, the area may be slightly massaged with a mixture of olive oil and grated garlic (2:1).

It is important to leave the injured part under cold water as often as possible.

varicose veins

The origin of most afflictions of the legs and veins is the slowing down of the circulation. A bad circulation is caused by rich and overcooked food, by overeating, and mixing all sorts of food at the same meal.

Nothing is more favorable to the restoration of a normal circulation than proper vegetarian food. The person should eat raw vegetables and fruits which are excellent blood fluidifiers, as often as possible. Garlic is especially good, because of the sulphured essences that it liberates in the digestive canal. Once absorbed in the interior walls with other elements created by the digestive process, these sulphured essences, gas included, are immediately absorbed into the blood which they help cleanse and fluidify. Moreover these essences exercise a cleansing action on the vascular walls, and a disinfecting one in any area that may be injured.

In order to fluidify and purify the blood, cleanse the vessels and normalize their flexibility, no toxic food may be taken, and strong food must be taken with care, especially concentrated food, which may deposit a layer of 'dirt' on the inside walls of the veins.

Whole wheat bread should be taken in moderation. Alternate it with rye bread. Make both whole wheat and rye bread with 85-90% sifted flour with a natural starter.

Cheese, dried fruits and most dried vegetables are to be drastically reduced since they are very concentrated. Also, food should not be cooked under too much pressure as it will be too concentrated.

Take herb teas good for the liver and circulation—plantain, persicaria, witch hazel, yarrow, cypress fruit, black currant leaves.

Dextreit recommends taking the following mixture of herbs after the third week of detoxification with fruits and vegetables: Hawthorn—20 gr; hyssop—20 gr; red-grape vine leaves—20 gr; shepherd's purse—20 gr; witch hazel —20 gr; yarrow—20 gr; matricaria (wild chamomile)—10 gr. Bring a pint of water to a boil and add 4 tablespoons of the plant mixture and steep for 15 minutes. Even better, let it steep overnight. Drink during the day, between meals.

Avoid local applications of clay in the beginning of the treatment. Clay is known to have the property of attracting all the toxins; do not give this part of the body an additional burden at this time. Premature applications may often create a swelling in the treated part. Complete the clay treatment with applications of raw cabbage leaves and later on with plantain leaves or Solomon's seal.

For large varicose veins, apply wet compresses dipped in an oak bark solution: 100 gr. of oak bark in a quart of water. Bring to a boil and let simmer a half hour.

As soon as this treatment produces a positive effect, start using the clay alone. Proceed simply with daubs of clay; that is to say, with the hand spread a good and uniform layer of cold clay paste over the greater part of the leg.

After 1 or 1½ hours, when the clay is dry, wash the leg and renew the daubs, if possible. Avoid very hot and thick poultices which could produce considerable drainage of toxic substances through the affected area. Light applications, repeated as frequently as possible, will yield good results with perseverance. At night, use a damp compress with a decoction of plantain or evergreen oak bark or a thin clay poultice, placing fresh plantain leaves or Solomon's seal on the top of the poultice.

Take cold hip baths every night before going to bed and upon waking up in the morning, for this activates the circulation.

Use a tub large enough to be comfortable. It is quite acceptable to use a bath-tub, but rest the feet on a higher object, for they must not get wet. If a cold bath cannot be tolerated in the beginning, start with lukewarm water only 2″ deep. Day by day, gradually lower the temperature one or two degrees, until a temperature of around 65° can be tolerated. At the same time, slowly add more water until the level reaches the fold of the groin. Make sure the body does not become chilled and that the room temperature is warm enough to be comfortable.

Taken regularly, the cold hip bath greatly aids the curative process.

wounds and cuts

If it is recent, put clay powder onto the wound, then cover it with a large cold poultice. Bandage firmly.

After this poultice, which should be kept in place for a maximum of 2 hours, wash the wound with salted or lemon-water; after that, apply a compress of clayish water.

If the existence of foreign bodies in the wound is feared, continue the clay poultices until there is no more doubt. All the foreign substances will be absorbed by the clay, and later found there. There have been many cases where foreign bodies that were impossible to extract surgically have been drawn out by clay.

When the state of the wound allows it, expose it to the open air in order to hasten its healing. Sometimes it is necessary to apply a dry dressing in order to avoid friction or any other contact. This dry dressing may stick to the skin and present difficulties in removing it. To avoid this, use the following antiseptic pack; peel an onion; take out a layer carefully and extract the very thin membrane that is between two layers of onion. Apply this pellicle directly onto the wound, which it protects and disinfects. Add the dressing and bandage. This precaution is also very useful for any kind of dry dressing in general, such as ulcers and sores.

Chapter 7
COSMETICS

Clay's invaluable properties make it an ideal base for skin care products. It helps tighten pores, tone skin and preserve its natural balance. Although most active in its virgin state, clay may be blended with other natural ingredients to become highly effective deep cleansing masks, toothpaste, shampoo, and even soap. You may mix your own cosmetics or buy them ready-blended. A reputable beauty and hygiene company in France, appreciating the value of clay in skin care, has formulated an excellent group of products using green clay—considered to be one of the most active of all. These clay-based toiletries have been widely used in Europe for over 10 years and are now available in the U.S.

deep cleansing masks*

Perhaps the easiest way to use clay is as a skin beautifier. When applied to the skin as a mask, oxidation and circulation are accelerated, defensive functions stimulated and body temperatures lightly raised. Thus clay acts rather like a light massage. In addition, clay, as with every natural product, is a balancer and revitalizer.

Mask Recipe

To mix your own masks, make a paste by adding ½ a glass of water, ½ a cucumber, tomato, or grape juice to clay powder. Apply thinly and uniformly all over face, back, or wherever you have over-oily or troubled skin. Leave the pack moist as long as possible to give skin flexibility with no sensation of tightness. Then allow to dry and rinse off.

A more soothing cosmetic cream can be made by mixing clay powder with olive oil, or you can use the French masks, ready-blended with pure olive oil and sweet almond oil.

Treat any unwanted growths or blemishes with clay. Apply very thickly on a pimple or wrinkle at night and leave until morning.

Wash irritated, pimply, grainy, or very delicate skin with clayish water, without soap, then rub it with the inside of a lemon-peel.

Under-eye sacs are very much relieved or even disappear with clay applications and complementary treatment of heart or kidneys, whichever is responsible.

shampoos*

Clay is excellent for regular hair washing as it has a natural acid pH that is similar to the skin. It is particularly recommended for a greasy scalp. To combat this, make a clear paste with water and apply as a shampoo. Leave on for at least ½ an hour and rinse off. The European shampoos contain olive oil and plant-based foaming agents to bring hair back to its natural lustre.

toothpaste*

One of the best natural toothpastes is clay, or a mix of clay and sea salt. Being so absorbent, clay is completely non-abrasive. It lifts off dulling film, removes mouth odors naturally, and acts as a gum stimulant.

soaps*

Blended with honey and olive oil, clay makes a very effective soap. It removes deep-seated grime, acts as a natural deodorant, and balances the skin. The added ingredients bring their own softening and soothing qualities for first class skin care.

clays

There are different types of clay. Raymond Dextreit generally recommends the green clay for drinking purposes. This same clay is also excellent for poultices. It is available at almost every health food store.

*Soaps, toothpaste and shampoos can now be purchased at all health food stores.

Green clay is usually used for drinking purposes. French and now American naturopaths recommend it. It is also good for other needs like poultices, plasters, masks, cuts, etc.

Rose clay is a very smooth type of clay which is mainly used for deep cleansing masks, body packs, smoothing roughened skin. French people use it for pimples.

White clay is a very fine powder for all talc purposes. It is an excellent deodorant. It is particularly good for 'sticky' feet and hands, and ideal for babies and diaper rash.

Chapter 8
BUYER'S GUIDE

Buying the needed kind of food and herbs should not be difficult now. Years ago it was so, when health food stores were a rare thing and only carried a few items.

Organically grown vegetables were always available, but always expensive. When you think about it, though, it is not really much more expensive than the ones sold on the regular market, since a small amount of the organically grown is far more satisfying in taste and in nutrition. People tend to eat a lot more vegetables when the taste is not there; they are trying to "catch" the true flavor of the carrot or cabbage.

If you find that vegetables, fruits, and grains are too expensive in a health food store, you might try to form a co-op (just a few families) and make a big order to the wholesaler; this can give you savings of up to 40% off the retail price—and that is a lot if your main food is vegetables, fruits, and grains. If you should buy grains in bulk, make sure to put them in a cold place otherwise they get wormy after two or three months, more or less, depending on the temperature. Always keep them tightly covered in glass or earthenware jars.

Powdered clay can usually be purchased in bulk at all wholesale clay potter supply houses. The type of clays these companies carry are not to be used internally. They are too rough. However, the following companies carry fine clays that are good for all purposes:

H. R. Enterprises, Inc.
P.O. Box 4321
Fullerton, Ca. 92634
(Desert Mineral clay)

The Herbalist
934 N. Western Ave.
L.A., Ca. 90029
(Volcanic Ash)

George Comfort Products
P.O. Box 742
Soquel, Ca. 95073
(West German clay)

P. & S. Mining Co.
P.O. Box 104
Worland, Wyoming 82401
(Pascalite—Big Horn Mountain clay)

Nevalite Products
Box 628
Verdi, Nevada 89439

All clay products, for cosmetic as well as medicinal purposes, may be purchased from health food distributors and health food stores around the country. However, the one company that carries the most diversified list of clay products is CLAY FRANCE. They have the famous French green clay, the rose and the white clay. They carry soaps, toothpastes of various flavors, skin care lotions, toiletries, deodorants, and masks. They have come up with a practical travel pack, a jumbo tube of green mud that can be used for almost everything—as a poultice and for burns, cuts, bruises, mosquito bites, skin rashes, etc. They even have band-aids, believe it or not.

The address is:

CLAY FRANCE
400 North Orange Drive
Los Angeles, CA 90036
Telephone: 213 937-3100

Their products are distributed by:

Eden Foods
701 Tecumseh Road
Clinton, Michigan 49236

They may be purchased at any health food store.

Chapter 9
CLAY IN PREGNANCY AND SURGERY

Pregnancy

Clay, in combination with a natural diet, is highly beneficial for the formation of the foetus and in the preparation for childbirth.

Take a regular daily teaspoon of clay for one or two weeks.

If the child is badly situated, do not hesitate to apply clay poultices on the belly. For the sake of prudence, it is preferable to apply it systematically during the last month of pregnancy. Also place tepid clay poultices on the lumbar region if pains appear.

Cold poultices applied on the stomach just after the childbirth will prevent all subsequent troubles (principally, the risk of infection) and is the best remedy for the imperfect elimination of the afterbirth.

Clay drinking favors nursing.

Post-operative Complications

Clay applications give the best results for the reabsorption of adhesions, healing and other post-operative complications. It is not necessary to act immediately after the operation, but one or two months later.

Begin with very thin poultices ¹/₂-1 cm.) leaving them on for at least two hours. Then gradually increase to 2 cm. thick poultices.

If poultices are well-tolerated and if they do not fall apart, dry quickly or cool, they can be left in place overnight. At first try cold clay, but warm it in a double boiler if heating does not occur rapidly after application.

Note: It is not possible to foresee exactly what will happen with clay applications, especially at first but in every case, there is a remarkable improvement, if not complete healing. As there are no dangers to fear, there is no reason to oppose giving it a try, even for an extended period of time.

Let us repeat: apparent inconveniences at the beginning do not represent any danger; on the contrary, it is a sign of the efficient and beneficial action of clay.

You must remember to precede the treatment with laxative teas, a fruit or lemon treatment, vegetarian nourishment, and the absorption of clay by oral route, in order to greatly reduce the amount of toxins in the organism. It is only after ten days of this preparation that clay treatment should begin.

For those who are not acquainted with clay, these affirmations may seem rather bold. How can a natural remedy as simple and cheap as clay perform such complex actions as: to void an abscess, to heal a cyst (even internal), relocate a badly placed foetus, help to rebuild destroyed tissues? How? No one knows. Those who would pinpoint it are bold indeed. Besides, the answer to this question is of but relative importance in the light of clay's effectiveness. We should be satisfied testing these powers. And so it is; more and more people are trying it every day, with very good results. Is this not the essence?